The Pioneers of
Interstitial Cystitis

PUBLISHED BY:

Norman Morrison

Facebook.com/NormanEMorrison

Copyright © 2015

Dedicated to the memory of Dr. Paul Fugazzotto Ph.D

Pioneers of Interstitial Cystitis

Introduction to Pioneers of IC

Thank you for purchasing this book. I presume that you have Interstitial Cystitis or know someone who does; else you would not be reading this. Rarely can anyone outside our sphere of friends even pronounce the name. Even we have trouble spelling it.

I say "we" because I have had IC since 1982. As you know, only one out of ten who develops the malady are male, and I'm definitely a guy. Don't let that put you off, however. I have spoken with a great many women who have it, so there isn't much I haven't heard.

The purpose of this book is to give a snapshot of what was going on with IC research during the golden age of *armchair urologists,* as I called them from 1988 to 1991. It is offered as a historical document. However, be advised that it is from the early labors and researches of these good people that much of the practical treatments of IC taken for granted today came from.

What you will find here is a reprinting of a volume of newsletters that I produced called **The IC Disclaimer.** It was not a pretty newsletter, or "magazette" as I called it. It was not scholarly. It often rambles. But it was unique and useful, as a clearing house for as much homespun information as I could find to report. At the height of its popularity it had, probably, a hundred fired up subscribers. I often used (or attempted) humor to give my readers a smile.

On the flip side, this book is not about the institutional researchers of IC. Those learned men and women who gathered millions of dollars over the years to do basic laboratory research. That is for someone else to extol and explain to what practical pain relieving purpose it ever served. Seems like the last time I checked the cause and cure of IC is still pretty much unknown.

This book is about the above average IC sufferers at home who added life saving IC knowledge, often by experimentation on themselves, rather than sitting around waiting for the lab coats with their test tubes, grinding along in their theoretical glacial ways.

A byproduct of this book is to remind or enlighten the reader that Interstitial Cystitis is the result of bacterial infection. This is something that has been known by the readers of the ICD and roundly ignored by the research community for at least twenty five years as of this publication.

Like the weather, IC has been studied for decades. It's still being studied. Unfortunately, rarely has anyone set out to do anything about it. You'll see some exceptions in this book.

There is a second purpose for this book. I knew way back that there might come a day when the newsletter files might come in handy. With the advent of self publishing, that day has come. The retelling of the ICD days is a bit of unfinished business with me. Now, I'll finish it!

The Author's Credentials

Long story short, I have had nothing less than a lifelong interest in science, natural curiosity, and an ability and desire to do research to educate myself on whatever interests me, and a very personal experience with interstitial cystitis. I am happily unlettered.

In 1982 I was a happy warehouse worker taking care of business and the family. Then one day while driving my forklift I noticed a pressure on my bladder, so I loosened my belt a couple of notches.

By and by I would have bouts of passing blood in my urine. Then, later, I would find dried blood flakes in the bowl. Frankly, it was just a curiosity at the time, since I was young, dumb, strong as an ox, and invincible. I was 27 years old.

But then, I started going down pretty rapidly. Because I had a young family and because I was stubborn, I refused to quit the hard labor which aggravated my condition. Many days I would go to work and at the end of the shift come home only to fall into the bed. It was about this time that someone called the "grass police" to come tell me that my front yard needed cutting. I just couldn't do it.

Thankfully, that year, I was in the first round of layoffs as the company got into a downsizing frenzy. Unfortunately, it was also about that time, without insurance, that I made up my mind to go to a doctor.

The old urologist was mystified. The first thing he did was to insert a large diameter metal probe up my penis to check for bladder stones. The old rascal never told me what he was about to do. He just grabbed and shoved. I'm still mad about that.

Undeterred, he set me up with a government "back to work program" that paid the freight for me to go to the prestigious UAB hospital in Birmingham, Alabama, so the urology department could diagnose my mystery disease.

After a couple of days of tests, that evening a wizened old urologist in a splendid lab coat breezed through with a bevy of students behind him, grinned broadly, and pronounced me fit as a fiddle, to be released the next morning.

About three that morning I was sitting up in bed smoking a Marlboro, puzzling over the non diagnosis when a young, skinny orderly, angel, something, strolled in and plopped down in the chair. After bumming a smoke from me, I told him my story. He shook his head and set me on a path that I follow to this day. He told me that sometimes there are no answers, so it was up to me to just make the best of a bad situation. Fight it.

After the fellow left, I sat pondering until the gray light of morning. I decided that I had contracted some kind of disease from Mars that nobody could figure out, least of all me. I decided the last thing I'd do was sit around and mope. So, stubbornly, I got on with my life, and tried to do it in a good humor.

Despite my bladder scarring and shrinking down to a walnut capable of holding no more than an ounce and a half at a time, and despite having to plan my life around toilets and bushes, many times no more than five minutes apart, I decided that I would fight, raise my kids, love my wife, and not let it lick me.

I must say that my immediate friends and family, who had to adjust around me, did it with more grace than I probably would have, had the shoe been on the other foot. Living with someone with IC is no picnic, especially if they are grouchy at times from the constant pain. Looking back, if the folks around me had been less understanding, with all that I had on me, I may not have succeeded in adjusting as well as I did.

As I was fond of saying, "If you're averse to pain or scared of urine, then you have the wrong condition."

Living with IC is not fun, but at times, it can be pretty funny. Like the time I had to run to the bushes at mid day, on a mall frontage, and my ride ran off and left me...in a strange town. Now that was funny. Thank goodness they had only circled back around on the busy big town mega highway to pick me up. They had a swell laugh on my account.

If you're like me, when you think back to places you have visited, unlike normal people, you have fond memories of restrooms. I still remember that hot, smelly, wonderful outside restroom at the airport in Manaus, Brazil. Nice!

The Disclaimer

Yes, IC can be humorous, as well as challenging, which brings me to the name of the newsletter presented on these pages. It was called **The IC Disclaimer**. Alright, you say, but why?

First, let me explain that at the time people did not sue each other wantonly, especially in my part of the country, Dixie. Just wasn't done. So, "disclaimers" were fairly foreign to me. I simply didn't see the need for them.

Yes, I know that today, especially if you just got off the last bus, this is tantamount to heresy. But trust me when I tell you that in 1988 it just wasn't common at all.

In 1988 there was an organization from up north, dedicated to IC, which was already well established. It was from them that I made contacts with people in their local chapters from which to peddle my magazette. I do not recall how I learned of them in the first place. This was a time before the Internet.

The organization I'm talking about will not be named. Henceforth, when referred to, it shall be called the XXX.

At the time, they struck me as real picky about their name. Second, they introduced me to the concept of the disclaimer. Well, me and everyone else. After they set the pattern nobody ever even said boo unless they started it off with a disclaimer.

Since 1991 I have not had any contact with them. I have purposely done little contemporary research on them, except to see that they are still around and still the 879 pound gorilla in the small restroom of IC. You can't miss them. They are that big.

This book is not about them. However, without them, there would have been no IC Disclaimer and no book. Whoever they are, they deserve a credit...but honestly, I don't know how to go about it without worrying that I will step on toes somewhere and they are the gorilla in the room, after all. It is enough to know that they exist, the organization that will not be named.

Quite frankly, any time you present something like the IC Disclaimer to the public there is always a risk. The XXX organization set the standard long ago when it came to minimizing risks. At the time I thought it was a complete hoot, and that's why I named my magazette as I did, as a humorous jab at all the disclaimer stuff out there.

Now, today, I see that the XXX organization was simply just ...ahead of its time.

But in 1988 I came to believe that the XXX organization was so dutiful in minimizing risk, that it failed to disseminate the research findings, anecdotal all, of their members. That's why the IC Disclaimer sprang to life as a niche publication to form a network of armchair urologists who were doing great, practical, every day work to make the lives of us sufferers more palatable until the lab coats came up with the cure. Which they never did, by the way.

Even though in 1988 I was not so dumb and unlearned as to understand that publishing what amounted to health opinions carried risk, I was determined to do just that, because it surely was not being done elsewhere. As such, it made me nervous. Still does.

Today, what you will read is history. At the time it was ground breaking and potentially life saving.

I beg of you to look on this as a window into the very foundation of IC self help by smart and courageous sufferers. Some gone on now.

If you find something in these pages you want to investigate yourself, it would be wise to do your own due diligent research among your fellow IC folks before attempting it. What you will read here may have been disregarded long ago. Remember, this is HISTORY...not current research.

And now, as the header promised, I give you the almighty disclaimer:

The IC DISCLAIMER and THE PIONEERS OF Interstitial Cystitis does not engage in the practice of medicine. It is not a medical authority, nor does it claim to have medical knowledge. In all cases the IC DISCLAIMER and THE PIONEERS OF Interstitial Cystitis recommends that you consult your own physician regarding treatment or medication.

Additional note: The ICD is terribly out of date. While many things we discovered are still useful to know, many other experiments led nowhere and were discarded. <u>This book is presented first and foremost as a historical document</u>, not an instruction manual. Common sense MUST be observed at ALL times.

Just ahead you will read my surviving copies of The IC Disclaimer. But first, a bit of information on the publication.

When the magazette was published, at every opportunity names and contact information was given.

Obviously, these many years later, the contact information is totally out of date. Some of the folks are in fact, dead. Because of privacy concerns, names and addresses have been redacted. In some cases, when I have been able to relocate them in the process of writing this book, with their permission, updated contact information is provided.

Regardless, the information they provided has been left intact, which is all that matters for posterity and historical accuracy anyway. You can't contact George Washington, for example, to verify what he had for breakfast before boating the Delaware River. That he did is enough.

It is interesting to note that the magazette itself was produced on a Commodore 128 computer in C-64 mode. I bought mine at Sears, but they were first available at toy stores. It had an internal memory of 32K which probably wouldn't suffice to print a (.) period on a modern machine.

Never the less, the magazette was written and even sported rudimentary graphics, which was mighty nifty for the time.

I don't 100% recall how I was able to actually save the files to something viewable today, but I believe that what I did was to open them on the C-128 and run the text over to someone else's computer using a computer bulletin board system (BBS). The text was then recorded to a PC floppy, which I saved until I was able to access it with my first PC.

Regardless, I do have the text portion of the newsletters here for your enjoyment, enlightenment, and as an all but lost portion of the history of IC investigation.

The files languished until 2002 or so when I stashed them on an early website that I owned. I never went to any work to make the files public, though anyone could see them if they knew they were there. At the time I made comments from time to time which I leave intact here. As I make additional comments for the book, I'll make sure that you know they are contemporary.

So, what you will find on the following pages is:

- The original IC Disclaimer.
- Comments from the 2002 version.
- Contemporary comments for the book version here.

The ICD was written with humor at times, but also with an eye to accuracy. Its easy going style was meant to set the reader at ease, and at the same time impart vital information to alleviate as much suffering as possible. Most readers, I think, looked forward to each issue.

I know you're worn out with all this introduction stuff. Now we'll get to the reason you purchased this book in the first place. I give you The IC Disclaimer! (And yet another introduction!)

Introduction to the IC Disclaimer opening comments circa 2002...

The Disclaimer:

(Editor note<2014>: This is the intro from 2002)

The ICDisclaimer was a "magazette" that was published from 1988-1991 and was at once a humorous offering about the condition known as Interstitial Cystitis, and a serious effort to disseminate information that was not being delivered to the IC patients then....Or since, I am afraid.

Although the little bi-monthly magazine has been gone for some time, the information it contained is only old if you have already seen it. If you have interstitial cystitis, you may be interested in revisiting selected excerpts from the ICDisclaimer, (so named as a jab at certain IC information organizations because of the lunatic insistence of that a disclaimer be attached to everything, even toilet paper that bears their name). You will no doubt find valuable insights into your health problems that will help you to make sense of your malady. The fact that you are here proves that you are researching your problem. Don't give up, answers are out there.

Keep in mind that some things presented below will be helpful; some won't, because each case of IC is unique. You must be the judge. Let your pain be your guide.

The motto of the ICD was, "If it hurts, don't do it." It is a good lesson for IC, it is a good lesson for life.

Many conclusions that were drawn by the ICD were and still are unsubstantiated by research, but that is not the fault of the ICD. No. It is the fault of the clinical money pits out there that have drawn millions from your taxes and produced nothing. The reason is simple; they stubbornly refuse to look in the right direction. They wouldn't know the truth of IC if it smacked them upside the head, as the saying goes.

I say this with sad confidence. The history of IC research supports this conclusion. On the practical side, your doctor is handicapped by the fact that he must treat you with the known. So much time and money has been wasted on esoteric research that may well never bear practical fruit that it fairly boggles the mind.

The ICD was written by a gentleman who suffers with IC. Me. I am not a doctor, paid researcher, or an opportunist. I offer you nothing but information. The ICD, and my journey into that valley ended in 1991, yet through the web, I see that I have one last chance to show you some of the things I, along with the help of my friends/readers, discovered along the way. I hope this helps.

(Editor note<2002>: I used to rail against the disclaimers ever present on anything to do with Interstitial Cystitis. It was one of the reasons I took pen and ink in hand and began the ICDisclaimer to begin with.

With hindsight, I can see now that the organization that started the disclaimer fashion, known hereafter only as XXX, was amazingly ahead of its time. You see, back then, people didn't bring suit against each other at the drop of a hat like they do today.

Today, however, it is only good business sense to wrap yourself with all the magical charms and legal disclaimers you can lay a hand to before going forth into the public.

Thus, be advised and warned as you read that if you try anything on yourself that you learn from these pages, or extrapolate on your own from the trial and errors below, as always, we never told you to do it. So, if you take a magic powder and get a tummy ache, don't come running crying back here. There are NO proven cures in this book. Whenever we experiment on ourselves, we have no one to blame or to thank for that matter other than ourselves. This must be stressed much more strongly now than just a few years ago.)

Now on to The IC Disclaimer...

The IC Disclaimer Issue 1

My name is Norman Morrison and this is the first issue of the IC DISCLAIMER. I trust that you will be patient as the format evolves in the coming months.

Since this is what I call a How ya'll doin issue in which we will get to know one another, I'll go ahead and brief you on the general makeup and make suggestions.

This little newsletter is your chance to speak up on IC. We want to know what you think. What are your theories on the subject? Have you found something that helps your IC?

The rest of us are dying to hear from you. In fact, if we don't hear from you I'm afraid we'll have a very short publishing history. Consider the IC DISCLAIMER as the Phil Donahue of the IC world.

Some topics to reflect upon include, of course, substances that have helped, theories on the cause and cure of IC, ways to motivate local doctors and urologists, success stories of all kinds, things we haven't thought of, things we should be thinking about. Share your experience and read about others.

—Did you know that many IC folks also have intestinal woes?—

For many of us, life with IC has been one big old disclaimer. When you first come down with it your local GP disclaims that you indeed have cystitis and loads you down with antibiotics. Later when you go to your area plumber (urologist) he disclaims that you have cystitis, (prostatitis if male) and God knows what all if you are female.

Since I'm a male I don't profess to know the secrets between woman and gynecologist, but they also disclaim one thing or another. Finally, you luck up on the right doctor, or read about yourself in a magazine, (SAY! THAT'S ME THEY'RE TALKING ABOUT IN THIS HERE ARTICLE!) and you join the XXX, and lo and behold, another disclaimer. I hope that the one on the top of this magazette is the last one you ever see.

I don't personally have a clue as to what causes IC. I'm not alone. The great learned minds of our time don't either.

I realize that some of you may be reading this at the Chicago XXX meeting.

(Editor note<2002>: Please note. When you see XXX, it is substituted for the initials of an organization that you will probably recognize if I left it intact. For several reasons, mostly their insecurity, I will not mention their name. As they say, information is power, and they were and still are the lord high mistresses of information. The ICD challenged their authority by providing all the information, a fact they did not take kindly to.)

(Editor note(<2014>: A bit of clarification. The ICD came about because at that time I perceived that XXX organization did not present enough *practical* survival information to their membership. The ICD was to be a clearing house of hints, tips, and experimental data from armchair urologists. The practical reason to NOT do this was of course the chance that someone would get sick from something that worked for someone else, and then there I would be. It was a little scary, a little fellow like me stepping out, taking chances, but I felt that helping people made it worth the risk. Common sense among my readers did prevail, and the ICD did no harm as it struggled to do good. It's even more scary today so you be sure you READ the disclaimer!)

Consider me envious. I urge you to develop some ideas and write to us about them. One thing that I do know firsthand is that you are what you eat, and eating has killed more people than all the wars the world has ever had. Many IC sufferers are hurting a lot more than necessary because of their diet. You may have food allergies, the meanest, hardest kind of allergy to track down and deal with. Something in that Pizza you had on Saturday night can lay you on your back Monday, and you could have felt great Sunday. This is my pet area and one that I'll come back to in future issues.

Unlike most of the things that afflict us, relatively little is known about IC, or perhaps as Mark Twain puts it, "Inflammation of the entrails."

I can't stress enough, the importance of sharing your thoughts and knowledge on the subject. Nearly everything we discover about IC breaks new scientific and medical ground. We may eventually give the scientists some new avenues to study. You may call the IC DISCLAIMER the magazine of IC Tips And Tricks. Survival is what we're all about until someone gives us a mighty pill to take care of our problems. What can you tell the rest of us that will help us get by?

The IC DISCLAIMER is published as a non-profit venture. It is not tax-deductible, so you can't bump Uncle Sam. It will be published 6 times within the coming year, and the cost is a buck an issue or $6.00 a year. It looks like an issue will cost between .50 and .70 cents to deliver to your door. The excess money will be kept in an uh-oh fund. My time is of course free. My payback will be the development of some hard information that can help us with our IC. Your check for a year's subscription will help. The magazette is being prepared on a Commodore 128 computer. If you have a C-128 or use GENIE services, please contact me. * * * * .

Thank You so much, and God Bless. Please write.

The IC Disclaimer Issue 2

This is the second edition of the Disclaimer. I'd like to extend a special welcome to our new subscribers. I get a heartwarming thrill whenever I get a letter and check in the mail from someone whom I don't know, but someone who enthusiastically wants and needs the services of this little magazette.

In case you missed the first issue, let me briefly explain the mission of the ICD.

For those of us who suffer with IC, there was a real information void. On one end, it seems that the XXX is primarily concerned with basic research, and on the other, our doctors have their hands tied and must use standard, tested treatments and medicines. We need and admire them both, but as we study our own conditions and communicate to others it becomes apparent that there is a lot of homegrown data out there.

The ICD serves as the clearing house for these new ideas, and a repository of knowledge that may prove helpful to the XXX and researchers. We are so used to giving our lives over to someone else it's tough to realize that sometimes we have to depend on ourselves. Sadly, some don't make the connection.

Case in point: Several months ago, I met a young lady over the phone that lives in north Alabama. She has a bad case of IC.

I discovered some things in my own life that eased my symptoms and I wanted very badly to share them with her. I wanted to share them with everybody, thus the ICD was born, because I realized I could go broke writing letters and using the phone. In my one on ones, I did find however that many of us who are prone to study our conditions have a lot of similarities.

Well, to shorten the story, I sent her a copy of the first issue and she wrote back, in part, "I will say that I can't believe that anything I eat makes my symptoms worse."

If you will recall, one of my main contentions is that what we eat can cause problems. Perhaps, in her case, food allergies play no part, but then again. . . . I have not heard back from her, and I'm assuming that she's not interested in the ICD. She periodically goes to the emergency room for morphine shots. I was pretty depressed about this. I appreciate your letters of encouragement.

* * *THE CASE OF LYNETTE SIGG * * *

Several months ago, on my way to discovery, I ran across an article in an inspirational magazine by this young lady. Although the piece was primarily concerned with her journey of overcoming pain, it read like a typical case of IC. It took some doing, but I finally contacted her by mail, in Australia! I still can't say for sure that she had IC, but her description read like a textbook case. She claimed that she had overcome it. One of her weapons was the herb Slippery Elm which you can obtain at any health food store. Her recommendation was two tablets three times a day with meals. I tried it myself, and for a couple of weeks I felt tremendously better.

Although it didn't affect the frequency it did nearly stop the pain. She stressed, however, that Slippery Elm only covers over the problems, and that only by going on an elimination diet can the cure begin. She gave me the titles of a couple of books, both by the same man, and would you believe that this author makes his home in Tennessee?

Following out my lead I contacted the fellow; Dr. Crook, and he told me a bit about his work. It seems that he is currently working on the assumption that the yeast known as Candida Albicans (Did I say that right?) which can infest the human gut produces toxins that can cause a heck of a lot of discomfort down there. If you have had your lower intestines nearly catch on fire, or been suffering from pelvic pain in that region, you know what I'm talking about.

Although he didn't seem to know much about IC, obviously the problems of Candida and food allergies can aggravate our IC. You see, what you eat can hit you immediately or 3 days later as it is processed and moved through the system. Further complicating the situation, there's not always a direct (Let me STRESS, in my opinion) correlation between what you eat and the symptoms.

According to Crook, sugary foods aid the yeast infection which in turn introduces toxins into the system. These toxins can make you have watery eyes, they can elevate your blood pressure, they can give you diarrhea, or none of the above. On the other hand, you can be directly allergic to a food, and as it moves through the tubes give you a whole range of problems, or maybe this times nothing. It's the darndest mess you've ever seen, but for many of us IC folks, it's our mess.

Lynette S., with the aid of a good allergy man said she overcame her problems. It might be a good area for us to look into. Keep in mind one thing. A lot of this ground has already been plowed ahead of you, to some extent. Sometimes it works and sometimes it doesn't. Two explanations are possible.

One: That's the way it is.

Two: Food allergy science is in its infancy and thus not well understood, and is not always applied correctly. I'll take theory number two. One other thing to keep in mind is that if you intend to pursue the food allergy route, be sure to use a doctor that subscribes to it. In my area at least out of the dozens of regular allergy doctors, only one, and he's 60 miles away in Birmingham advertises that he treats food allergies.

I'm afraid that even in this day and age food allergists sometimes get put into the category of chiropractors and urologists that treat IC. You may write for information on Crooks books at <Address> You may be able to find his book, TRACKING DOWN HIDDEN FOOD ALLERGY. If they don't have it they may be able to get it from another library for you. I'll shush on this subject by saying that it got me to thinking. I tracked down my number one unknown allergen; the one that put me in the hospital; fresh tomatoes. Yep. I figure it was the seeds. You wouldn't believe the difference. Of course, tomorrow I might become allergic to something else, but at least I'll have a weapon. Knowledge.

***IN THE MAIL ***

FROM Melanie B: (**Editor note<2002>:** - Please note here that I will shorten all the names to protect the privacy of the people who contributed to the ICD. In the original text the full names as well as addresses and phone numbers were used in most cases. The prospect of placing this material on the web was not even an idea at that time.)

Melanie writes that Arta C, the (XXX) State Coordinator read an excellent book called CANDLES IN THE DARKNESS by Amy Carmichael. She said it helped her. Melanie reports that Dixie K, (Enjoyed chatting with her a couple of weeks ago) wrote that a bladder instillation of DMSO/Heparin/Kenalog made her pain free. I hope she's still holding. I'll let you know, if I hear from her.

Dixie also reports that low acid tomatoes help. For sure, you can find them in most seed catalogs. Minute Maid markets a low acid orange juice for your palate. Also recommends a vaginal lubricant called Astroglide. You might also check out Serenity Pads by Johnson & Johnson.

Dixie recommends the book, YOU DON'T HAVE TO LIVE WITH CYSTITIS by Larrian Gillespie.

An interesting note: I found out about IC through an article by her in an obscure little science magazine. I breathlessly rushed to my urologist and showed him the article.

"I've got IC!" I said. He said, "Naw, you have arthritic bladder." Hmm. Sound familiar? It took me two more years, but I finally was diagnosed as NOT having arthritic bladder, whatever that is.

* * * * * CONSIDER: You have good days and bad days, right. Something changes. Find that something and we'll be close to the solution of the IC riddle! ********************************

MORE RULES?! Here's how you can help thee and me: Keep those letters coming, particularly if something you see in these pages is similar to your condition. There is strength in numbers, particularly if they add up to a statistical curve. Next, when you write, if in longhand, print very plainly any medical terms or product names. You may remember the one about the patient who when asked by their gynecologist how the spermicidal foam was working said it was working great but tasted terrible. We have to get those terms right. It is perfectly OK to make sample copies to give to friends, doctors, and so forth, but please ask them to subscribe.

One of my goals is to build a large enough base so that we can conduct real polls to see what we have in common with our IC. That's why I need them on roll. By all means help me enlarge this work any way you can. Get your group and state leaders to come on board. Also, if any of you have contacts in the western half of the nation, by all means introduce them to the ICD. This is a grass roots effort that will only succeed if everybody uses whatever influence they have to help it along. Also, remember that the form of this mag is fluid. I'm all for suggestions for improvement!

The IC Disclaimer Issue 3

(**Editor note<2014>**): At some point in the transfer process the division between issues became unclear, so at times I'm guessing where one left off and the next begins. Regardless the text that remains is all here.)

* * * IN THE MAIL * * * A super letter from Jan J down in Corinth Miss. . . . . . She writes, "From what you said about foods I thought you might have read some of Dr. Sherry Rogers books—"The E.I. (Environmental Illness) Syndrome.

She asks, "Are you allergic to the 21st Century?"

Well, no, I haven't read the book, but I'll be down to the library shortly to see about it. I think that about sums up IC. It just goes to show that IC folks here and there and over yonder are coming to the same conclusions independently, about the causes of their problems. The ICD hopes to tie them together. Thanks Jan, and God bless you.

Also thanks Judy P from Killen Al. We'll be looking forward to hearing more from you.

* * * * Just a short take. I hastily scribbled down an address from a Donahue segment the other day. It seems like there is yet another group out there called P.A.R.F. (Beats me)<Address> who are working on food allergies.

It seems that there are kids out there who have been diagnosed as being hyperactive and treated with drugs when their problem is really food allergies. These people are actually giving them allergy injections made from food substances and its working. One kid was even pronounced autistic. Removing milk from his diet fixed him right up. They probably don't know much about IC, but the allergy shots (I have been told this is very uncommon in the field) may be worth following up on.

They say that all allergy doctors don't believe in their treatments. Sound familiar? I invite you to follow up on this and report your findings about how this can help to the ICD. Make letter in care of Doris R. with P.A.R.F. *
*

(**Editor note<2014>**): Doris Rapp is still busy as of 2014. I received a note from her assistant in reply to a FaceBook note that I sent. She is as insistent as ever of her allergy theory. You can reach out to her here: http://www.drrapp.com/ .)

I've had great success with DITROPAN 5mg tablets. I only take them when I have a bad flare up, preferring to hold control through diet. In case you're wondering, my bladder capacity couldn't be more than 1.5 ounces so even at the best of times 15 or 20 minutes is my limit. Well, anyway, I decided to call up the manufacturer, Marion Scientific. After a quick trip to the library and a look at the PHYSICIANS DESK REFERENCE, (A good book to know,) I gave them a buzz. After a while I got a young lady. I visualize her sitting there in a pristine environment with stacks of reference manuals. (**Editor note(<2014>**):According to Wikipedia Marion Merrell Dow and its predecessor Marion Laboratories was a U.S. pharmaceutical company based in Kansas City, Missouri from 1950 until 1996. It has since been acquired by another company.)

I asked a simple question...."Tell me about Ditropan. How was it developed? Who did it. When."

Ah, readers, the young lady was speechless. To make a long story short, she didn't know who invented it or how. It seems that their company evidently picked up the process from unknown sources and started making the stuff. She could have told me how it's supposed to work, but I got info from the PDR. Things have gotten so complicated out there that without extensive checking that particular lab didn't even know where they got the drug. (**Editor note(<2014>**): Or at least the lady on the phone didn't.)

This is NOT to say that they don't know their business, they just forgot their history. My question dealing with the development of drugs was never answered. Who said that going to the top was always best? I did find out in an ensuing phone call that Ditropan was developed some 20 years ago and is not marketed for use with IC. The reason. . . .Very little is known about IC so no research in that area was done, therefore the FDA hasn't approved the label to read thus, even though the makers know that it is being used for that purpose.

I'm sure that our other drugs also fall into this trap. This sounds like an issue to be pursued in a later edition.

*Many thanks to Melanie and her newsletter.

* * * * I had an interesting chat with D. at the XXX home office in New York, (My wife Vicky cuffed my ear when she got the phone bill) the other day. She recommends the book "LIVING WITH CHRONIC PAIN, By Cheri Register, The Free Press. She also offered a couple of tips. First, a note from the doctor may get you quicker admittance to some event if presented to a sympathetic ticket seller.

Second, it is possible that you could qualify through your doctor for one of those handicapped stickers to go on your car so you can park in the choicest spots. Now, by golly, many of us have a real need to go to the front, fast, so if you are of a mind, feel no shame! If IC isn't handicapping, I don't know what is.

D. also mentioned that one of our state folks nearly got nailed a while back because someone tried a course of treatment they recommended in a newsletter, without the ever present disclaimer, and got worse.

The reader blamed the state person for her added discomfort. D. might have remembered that I said one time that the XXX is paranoid about disclaimers. Well, they are, but with good reason. Remember, you have to use that good old common sense anytime you embark on a new course of treatment. Always preface your reading here with an..."In my opinion."

The IC DISCLAIMER does not engage in the practice of medicine. It is not a medical authority, nor does it claim to have medical knowledge. In all cases the IC DISCLAIMER recommends that you consult your own physician regarding treatment or medication.

OK. We are in hopes that D. can get clear to get us some state coordinators names to contact with the XXX (Never happened! Editor) and I believe that the ICD and the XXX have a good future together. I believe we are thinking along the same lines. Thanks D.!

* * * Please remember to P R I N T those drug names. * * *

Another super letter from super supporter Jan J. Jan writes that Kyolic Garlic capsules and chicken bullion help to relieve her IC. (See here, here's an example of common sense. I'm deathly allergic to onion products, although I don't think it directly affects my IC like some other foods, except for a generally screwed up G/I tract. I can't take garlic, but maybe you can. We've heard about garlic elsewhere, specifically from Crooks allergy books I think.)

She says that she tries to stay away from acid foods too. (Personally, I know that acid conditions aggravate IC, but I think there's more to acid foods and IC than their acid content. I believe in many cases that there is some unknown ingredient at fault. Read on.)

Jan mentions that she stays away from foods high in Oxalic acid. (A new one on me, but one I'm going to check into. I theorize that tannic acid is my main nemesis, and others of our clan have said as much, independently.)

She also uses DMSO/hydrocortisone. Jan says that it helps to stay as busy as possible doing things that are enjoyable, and to eat well. She is a Christian and doesn't hesitate to mention the source of her strength. I'm really glad to hear this. A great source of comfort can be found in your local church or through the mail with publications like Unity.

Jan wants to hear from girls who have had their bladders removed. She knows 3 girls who have Koch pouches. Also, and most importantly, she is conducting research into vulvular pain, extreme irritation and sensitivity. (I don't think I have one.)

She says that the bladder, urethral and vulvular pain come on at once and she believes they are connected. Please write her if you have some personal experience to contribute. I'm sure Jan will keep me posted on her progress. Write her at (X). * * *

Jan recommends: The E.I. Syndrome by Dr. Sherry Rogers, <Address>. It's about environmental illnesses.

My problem is sitting. A couple of years ago I got to where it is painful to sit on all but the softest surfaces for any length of time. I'd like to hear if this is common with any of you. Thanks so much for Jan's comments. Get in touch with her on this important subject.

    * * * -*-*-*-*-*-*-*- The IC Disclaimer is non-profit, but not tax deductible. One year costs $6.00. It is published 6 times a year. Please make your check payable to: (X) Back issues are available at regular price. Write.THANKS!

The IC Disclaimer Issue 4

Sheila N. Sheila was the first person I talked to about IC. I'm not exactly sure what her current status is in the Alabama IC hierarchy at present, but I will say that she organized the original effort, and at the very least helped the effort to become perpetuating.

Her contribution to IC is not so much information as attitude and influence. Her struggle symbolizes that which we have all had. She has really had some bad experiences with doctors and has fought the policy of removing the bladder as a first resort, which to my understanding is more common in Birmingham than may be necessary.

She recommends reading the book, "WHAT YOUR DOCTOR DIDN'T LEARN IN MEDICAL SCHOOL AND WHAT YOU CAN DO ABOUT IT! By Stuart M. Berger,M.D., Morrow 1988.

The average for getting properly diagnosed for IC in this country is 6 years, we're told, and I'm pretty average. I am extremely thankful that I found a good urologist.

When I first went to him I said, "I've got something you probably don't believe in."

He said, "Try me."

I said," I have IC."

He smiled and said, "If you've got it, I'm your man."

It took 4 years to find him. Sheila is convinced that her IC is due to a thyroid problem which she inherited, and is pursuing that avenue. I know that she will keep us up to date on her search for answers. Thanks Sheila.

D. at the XXX recommended a young lady to the mailing list. Valerie Z makes her home in New York state.(Do I type with a southern accent, Valerie?) I'm sort of tickled with her letter because she says flat out, "Because I have always believed in the body's basic ability to renew and restore its balance, I chose not the path of medical science."

Well, that sort of rules out Ditropan. I have to take exception to that philosophy, I wish I didn't, but we report all the news. Valerie says that she "Went through all the usual hysteria associated with being diagnosed properly with IC," which is a turn of phrase that I'll cherish and use in these here pages in the future.

The meat of Valerie's communication is her relationship with her doctor, Alfred Z. He is a dermatologist, allergist, and clinical ecologist. She says that he treats each person as a whole being,(where you live, what you eat, where you sleep, etc.)

Playing devils advocate a moment, Valerie says that Dr. Z's program is unique. I don't think so.

Dr. Crook in Tennessee is pioneering in the elimination diet area and I'll bet that book, the E.I. Syndrome gets onto his turf a bit.

Bear with me, I'm coming to a point in a little while. Valerie teased me a little. If you remember, last issue I said I thought I was allergic to tomato seeds. She says that many environmental factors and foods can cause hypersensitivity. Absolutely! She and my wife for that matter are allergic to fowl and eggs.

I have developed an allergy to eggs over the last couple of years. (I wonder if it's something in the eggs, antibiotics for instance, and not the eggs or chicken we can't take.) She says she's allergic to wheat germ, but can eat white flour. Does anyone out there have problems with pastries and cakes, but not white bread?

Valerie says that one lady she introduced was facing imminent bladder removal, but after being treated by Dr. Z was a "new person."

The lady is pain free and urinating less frequently. Dr. Z has a book out called,"WHY YOUR HOUSE MAY ENDANGER YOUR HEALTH".

Frankly, I wished I had the money to go see this man. Although he doesn't have the market cornered on allergies and IC, he seems to be our kind of guy. The point I was coming to is that from Valerie's description he seems to have tied several allergy technologies together to come up with a helpful program.

This is in no way a recommendation on my part, but it does sound extremely interesting for a lot of us. Should you wish to contact the good doctor Valerie was kind enough to include her address and phone number. Contact this young lady for information. Valerie Z, (X).

She's very interested in your allergy related endeavors, and we are darn well interested in hearing more from her! Keep the ICD posted on your efforts by all means! Thanks Valerie.

* * * Mail is the lifeblood of this magazette * * * The editor makes no bones about it. When you can, please introduce your friends and neighbors to the ICD and ask them to subscribe. This is an important work for the future of IC research. Thanks!

Lastly, let me introduce one of our newest subscribers, Dixie K of Mississippi. Dixie says to leave oats alone. I heartily agree. As a former Little Debbie Oatmeal Cake scarfing champion it was a bad day when I finally decided to lay them down. What's good for average folks can play havoc with the IC'ers of us. This is not to say that oatmeal products are necessarily bad for you, but Dixie and I can't have it so. . . . .

Actually Dixie has a whole lot more to say, so much so, that with her permission, I'm going to republish something she sent called, THE INTERSTITIAL CYSTITIS FACT SHEET, in the next newsletter. It is chock full of good information and should be kept within reach. Oh yes, Dixie relates that she too can't tolerate wheat bran. Hmm.

I realize that money may be tight for some of you, it is for us. I hope that you really find your money well spent with the ICD. The next issue is due to hit the stands in mid February. God Bless. See you next time.....Norman * * *

The IC Disclaimer Issue 6

The other day I chanced to meet my old urologist and friend Dr. H down at the lawnmower shop. Well, he was only slightly better humored at whiling away his time at the repair facility than me, but I did try, as best as I could to corner him and preach a bit of IC.

This, of course, placed me in the position of pupil trying to teach the professor. I'd tried that before in elementary school with a decided lack of success. As we parted, I offered to send him a copy of the ICD. Heck, I thought, why not fix it so everyone can have an issue to give to their favorite medical man? To follow is some fun facts to know and tell about Interstitial Cystitis.

IC is a so called syndrome that affects both women and men...about 90/10. Generally speaking it can occur any time after puberty, though in my experience it happens after age 25. There is only one recognized test for IC, and that's dilating the bladder with water and observing the results.

Every other tool and method commonly used in diagnosing regular cystitis can safely be left in the drawer. Question: How can you tell the difference between regular cystitis and IC?

Answer.....If after your regular research has failed to turn up anything, and urine cultures which may or may not contain infection fail to culture out an organism, then you may suspect IC.

People who have IC have been described as MULTI-SUFFERERS. Ladies and gentlemen differ in their problems on in only two significant areas. Women tend to develop vulvular pain, whereas men sooner or later show symptoms of prostatitis.

They may not actually have this problem, but the symptoms are the same. A super indicator of IC is that many have colon trouble. It is not clear at this time whether we actually do have a bona fide problem, but again, the symptoms are the same as someone with very tender innards.

Food is a major problem. For the IC afflicted, just about every healthful food can pose a risk. The problem can be two-fold. First, the lower intestinal area is or seems to be extremely sensitive, secondly, offensive products can transfer their poisons the whole time they are in the system to the scarred bladder causing a most intense pain. Here, let me show you a list of suspects.......

All alcoholic beverages(some late harvest wines excepted), apples, apple juice, cantaloupe, carbonated beverages, cherries, chili spices, cumin, ginger, Hungarian paprika, chutney, curry,citrus fruits, coffee, cranberries, grapes, guava, lemon juice, papaya, peaches, pickles, watermelon rind, persimmons, pineapple, rhubarb, pomegranate, strawberries, tea, tomatoes, vinegar, avocados, bananas, beer, brewers yeast, canned figs, champagne, cheese,('ceptin processed cheeses such as Velveeta, ricotta, mozzarella, cream cheese, string cheese, and cottage cheese.), chicken livers, chocolate,('ceptin carob or white....((maybe)), corned beef, eggplant, fava beans, lima beans, mayonnaise, NutraSweet, nuts, onions, pickled herring, prunes, raisins, rye bread, Saccharin, sour cream, soy sauce, Worstershire sauce, yogurt, and some vitamins...............

As if this list weren't enough, foods that are similar to any of the above can also pose problems.

If you have an allergy to lemon juice, for example, be wary lemon pie as well. You may also add environmental hazards such as pollens, dust, fungus,(like A/C airborne varieties) and the like. Possibly, one of the greatest things that you as a physician can do is to make your patients aware of this list. Many IC sufferers are literally eating themselves to death. You will not find this problem so defined and commented in any medical work.

My personal method for identifying gastronomic culprits is to first make a list of what I eat the most. One at a time, I'll lay off a food for a week or so and see what happens. If I feel better, I'll go back and eat a bait (Southern for whole lot) of it. If I feel worse, I'll repeat the process a couple or three more times. It's a long, hard, and continuous process. New allergies pop up seemingly overnight.

A rule of thumb with IC is that IC and allergies is a function of IC severity. The more severe the IC, then likewise the number and severity of the allergenic response. The response, by the way, is the intense burning and pain in the bladder and colon, with possible side effects associated with regular allergy like swelling, sneezing, etc.

IC comes in stages. At first, the victim may only complain of a pressure on the bladder. Maybe they think they have a hernia. By and by there comes burning at urination, and then frequent urination. By degrees, IC tightens its grip and the sufferer has to get up in the night. Eventually, as the pain sets in, an end stage IC'er may have to go to the can 100 or more times a day.

With cystitis, frequency is a dead giveaway. It is the same with early IC, however as it becomes more severe it is a good idea to switch the thinking over to how much urine is made per trip rather than how often. After drinking a quart of Gatorade an end stage IC'er may have to urinate 25 times per hour.

In reality, she may only be dropping an ounce and a half of fluid at the time. Scarring can occur in other places besides the wall of the bladder. By the time you see a person with undiagnosed IC, she may have been to a half-dozen physicians without success.

Some can handle it, some can't. You can do a great deal to brighten their life by telling them what they have. The national average to diagnosis in this country is 3-5 years. IC is tough all the way around.

YOU TOO CAN BE FAMOUS....Its easy and fun! The NIH has money allocated for IC research. The last time I spoke with them, they had more money than researchers. There are many novel and productive areas to be looked into, just waiting for the right person to jump in. It might be you!

We'll be happy to give you our ideas......just mention it! IC'ers are lucky to have a nice national network of fellow multi-sufferers with which to chat.

Foremost in the East is the XXX out of New York. You may write to me for details. They can be put in touch with folks like themselves in or close to their area. You know how beneficial this can be.

Of course, there is this little magazette. You'll find stuff in here that you just can't get elsewhere. Men even have a sub-group getting underway at this writing out of Canada. Just lately, an independent researcher has turned over some impressive findings. He has developed a new method of culturing urine and has identified a strain of bacteria that he says is common to IC patients. Early results show promise.

He is quite reasonable. He only asks for enough money to mail out his specimen bottle! If you would like to contact this gentleman, write or call: Paul Fugazzotto, <Address>(<**Editor 2002**>:This address is not current. Please check his address toward the end of this article. Even then it may be out of date. This is unfortunate if true. Dr. Fugazotto will be mentioned many times later on.)

Finis...... Please accept my thanks for reading this. Reaching doctors is tough sometimes. I would certainly appreciate any advice or help you might be obliged to offer.

The IC DISCLAIMER is non-profit, but not tax deductible. One year costs $7.00. It is published 6 times a year. Please make your check payable to: Norman Morrison, the editor of this magazette. Back issues as available are at regular prices.(The ICD ceased publication in 1991. Editor 2002)

Write. THANKS! All correspondence is considered public unless you specify otherwise. Your address may be made available to others with similar interests unless you say otherwise.

The mail has been a trifle light this round. The ICD is not offended. Here, lately, it too has been reduced to summertime speed. The speed at which new issues are released is a combination of factors; time, how much the editor feels like sitting down, and so forth. However ...found in the bag.......

Allan W, Co-coordinator of the XXX, Canada, sends his form greetings and announces that he's forming a little XXX sub-group called THE STANDING COMMITTEE. It's an inside joke, of course, that most guys with IC have a bit of a problem sitting down. Something in the prostate area goes to sleep and we experience some of that exquisite pain that is the IC trademark. Allan invites your ideas and support. I guess he'll let us know more later.....Write—Allen W.... I believe postage from the U.S. there is something around 45 cents, so best to slather up two stamps for your letter.

One of the kickingest groups around, that of Ruth K, in or around Fairfax Va, reports that they have heard that Dr. Fugazzotto had arterial surgery on his leg on August 14th. I know it must have been successful, because I've heard from him since. You can't keep a good man down!

*By the way.....I need to have some reports from those of you who have been experimenting with Dr. F.'s regime. I know that you want to wait around awhile before passing judgment...but all I want to know is how it is going or gone so far. Please let me hear your to date results, feelings etc...

Well, guys... Ruth K. reports that one of the Va. men has been diagnosed as having bladder cancer. She reports his name as Tom.......Tom was scheduled to have his bladder out on August 25. As Ruth pointed out in her newsletter, women don't have this problem too much, but men do, so fellows, protect yourself!

Your doc does have tests to indicate whether or not you coming down with the big C. I don't want to put another monkey on your backs...God knows we have enough, but do get a check every few months....I do! Good luck Tom!

From Wisconsin comes news of Holly. Remember, Holly had her bladder out a couple of months ago? I talked to her a while back and she asked me to express her thanks to all the ICD readers who sent cards and letters.

Alice J., super ICD supporter talks to her quite frequently. I might suggest that a little later, when Holly gets fully back onboard, those of you who are considering having your bladder removed contact Holly and ask her about the ins and outs of the procedure.

Betty L W of Florence, new mistress of the Alabama Gang wrote and sent a check. She reports that she has been invited to go talk to a whole hospital full of doctors about IC. I'll sure be interested in reporting how that came out! Sounds like a dream come true. I'm a might envious.

I'm tickled to report that two new coordinators came into the fold. Carol B writes from Delaware. We'll hopefully be hearing some good things from that corner of the country soon. Audrey H sends her regards from Marco Island, Fl. An Island? C'mon now..... Visions of palm laden beach bathrooms spring to mind.....

Audrey is an amateur IC researcher in the best traditions. She reports that she tried 300mg of Tagamet 4 times a day and it worked for a couple of months before it lost its effectiveness. She also gave an antihistamine called Hismanal a shot and said she had a strong bad reaction. She indicates that while Tagamet seemed to work fine, she's typically ICD semi-skeptical till further proof comes her way. She tells us to "Keep on a-smiling." I'm looking forward to hearing more from paradise.

Frank W signs on from Hernando, Ms. He's 51 and a former Greyhound Bus Driver and is currently a letter carrier. My first instinct is to say that Frank's case is non-typical, however, who am I to say what is and is not typical of a problem with so little research.

His letter raises questions but also sheds some much needed light on men with IC. Frank says that since '71 or '72 he has experienced some bladder problems. He says that for quite some time he could go for 4 hours at a stretch unless he imbibed of coffee or cokes. He says that in the day he does pretty good but has to go every hour or so after bedtime.

He says that he's going to give Elavil a try. Frank says that he doesn't have the bad pain associated with what I call end-stage IC. Since he's had it so long, perhaps he's stabilized before hitting the bottom. He says that it seems like each time a cysto was done (thrice) his frequency would increase. In trying to relate what I've heard, and myself to Frank, I can recall that my IC seemed to take 3 or 4 quantum leaps in 4 years or so before I bottomed out,(end-stage).

Frank seems to be at stage 2 or so. He says that he has tried (well kinda) laying off cokes and chocolate without being able to tell much difference. As I said earlier, as your IC moves through its stages, you progressively get allergic to more foods and substances. I theorize again...)

Ah, I remember a time when I'd scarf up a half-quart of chocolate milk and a sheaf of powdered doughnuts, not so long ago. Frank writes a very nice and informative letter. I am sure that you will be very interested in seeing how Frank progresses. Thanks!

Maybe it would be a good time to try and come up with an IC PROGRESSION CHART. You know that you just didn't wake up one day and, boom, there it was. What do you think? Would this be an interesting area to work on? In your mail, let me know as fancy or as simply as you like how you progressed to your current level. I'll put them all together, shake well, and pour out a report......

JUST FOUND! I believe it was Jan J down in Ms. that first reported on the Environmental Illness Syndrome. Well, I just received a newsletter from the ALLERGY & EI SUPPORT GROUP OF ALABAMA <Address>It is a state group, much like the XXX and its little chapters. Since the ICD takes so much to heart from the EI movement, (Stuff around you makes you sick) I am pleased to give you this address. They publish 4 times a year, and though supposedly mostly concerned with Alabama, send their paper all over the place. I had a chance to speak at length with Gail B, their state coordinator. I think their organization could teach ours a lot. I told her that IC'ers are allergic to just about everything that is considered good and wholesome, possibly even Wilford B. and his oatsies. (<Editor 2014>: A clever aside to actor Wilfred Brimley who was hawking oats at the time.)

She said she'd be tickled to hear from my readers, who'd like more info. At any rate, I'm sure that you'll be hearing more about them, as time and space allow. (<Editor 2014>: I spoke with Gail. She's still around and helping folks with her wisdom as of 2014!)

* If its new, theoretical, or just different, you're probably going to see it in the ICD. You may often find in the pages of the ICD, proof that you are not alone in your thinking on IC. Many folks, separated by many miles have come to the same conclusions, independently, about their condition.

Since, so very little hard research is available, we just don't have time to apply the traditional scientific method to our problem. Until it comes along, the best we can do is to compare notes and see what we come up with. If you have hard research to report, please do so. Likewise, if you just think that you've noticed a pattern to your IC, let the rest of us know. Little things are important! Say, if you were able to go to the last XXX convention, and have some notes to pass along for those of us who didn't attend, I'll be happy to get them in the next ICD. * * * * * *

The art below was contributed by a non-IC type.... (Should we make him an honorary IC victim?) by the name of Jimmy P. Thanks James! I want to express my thanks to my friends in Ga. & WS. who have allowed me to stretch out with extra issues in my colonization efforts.

It's paying off. I must mention that this magazette is actually a bi-partisan effort. I do the master-minding, but wife Vicky gets it copied and mailed.(She hates my computer.)

Speaking of computers....this mag is done on a Commodore, and is available directly from the phone lines, (your dime.) Oops. This is this is issue #6, so the next round starts with the next one probably sometime in late October or November. (I'm a month behind, but catching up....)

It's to re-up with 7 bucks to get 6 more issues of fun facts to know and tell about your chosen illness! If you haven't already done so, make your check payable to me soon.

Your mail, of course, is what the ICD is all about. Your research and experiments are vital to the rest of us.

THE IC DISCLAIMER
THE BIMONTHLY NEWSLETTER FOR INTERSTITIAL CYSTITIS
YOUR EDITOR: NORMAN MORRISON
THIS MONTH: "A NEW PATH?"

IC has been recognized in one fashion or another since the turn of the century. By and by, tight little knots of researchers have added their knowledge to the cause. Mostly, their efforts were too little, and probably received the same amount of attention that modern researchers are used to. That is to say, very little.

Some of their "discoveries" are still with us today, and being used by some physicians who, having little to go on rely on the sparse leavings of their ancestors. Some of these treatments were used by young Frankenstein. Some of them have been used on some of you. One place sticks out in my mind particularly. It is at the summit of what I always considered to be the end of the line for men of good will, humanitarianism and knowledge.

Quite frankly, if some of the treatments that have been described to me were to be performed on a monkey at this world famous clinic, I suspect Cleveland Amory and his animal friends would seek an injunction. No doubt, at the very least, the animal would not survive. This but touches the very outer layers of my disgust for certain medical practices where IC is concerned.

OK, my venom level has been sufficiently reduced to proceed. As you know, the ICD preaches less is better than more. This is not to say to you, don't seek the best medical advice you can find. Just use a little common sense along the way.

Unfortunately, most readers of the ICD already know this, having been through the fires of silly treatments. It is the paradox of the illness. The folks who need information the most are the least likely to get it. They don't know about the ICD yet. They don't know about the XXX, and they don't know about your support group.

As you know, they'll stumble around for 3 to 5 years before they find out about us. I did it. You probably did. This is one area that has us boggled. Until some famous politician or good looking movie star gets a good case of IC, we'll just have to do the best we can to spread the word.

Age breeds patience. Ah, I am the modicum of patience, or so I thought. A few weeks ago I was gnawing the fat with Melanie B, the SE XXX coordinator. I told her that a certain individual had proven a disappointment to me. This individual had some big ideas that never seemed to go anywhere.

Melanie, being a third smarter than me, said a simple thing....

She said, "Well, maybe said person doesn't feel like carrying thru with the project just right now. Said person has IC, you know."

Woof. Right there, she had me. I'm only a couple of months late getting out the ICD. I'll flat tell you that half of this thing will be typed with me standing up. (That's a man thing...) I just had to tell you about that one.

As a matter of fact, Melanie, that mountain of strength, who I look to for IC inspiration told me some things about Melanie....some of her problems. It only makes her that more dear. Most of the time, a person who has been blessed with IC just doesn't have time for patience in some areas. Let us always remember to have patience with ourselves...Right, XXX corporate?

Alright.... Now..... Let's launch into a little history lesson in preparation for what could prove to be the news of the decade in IC...maybe. Early this summer, it must have been, I found out about a gentleman by the name of <Dr. Paul Fugazzotto>who had some unique ideas about IC. Again, the wellspring sprung in Melanie B's newsletter. It seems like he made a big XXX meeting early this year. I talked to him the same day Melanie's letter arrived, although, at that time, after spending nearly an hour on the phone, I was still mostly in the dark.

Time moves on...I tried his approach to the treatment of IC, and so did some others. I think I mentioned him in the last two ICD's, although cautiously. Caution, not so much from the standpoint that I feared some sort of scam...more so, because I was waiting to hear from others who had tried his cure.

Frankly, I'm still waiting for more feedback. Those of you out there who are sitting around waiting to hear what everybody else has to say ought to get on with it. But, here I start to meander. October 9th rolls around..... <Dr. Fugazotto> attends a meeting organized by the Virginia IC'ers. What follows is a verbatim portion of Ruth K's newsletter. Ruth and her bunch is in the forefront of amateur IC research these days, and enough good things cannot be said about her.....

Here, read on...

Here at last is my report to you on our meeting with on October 9th. A delightful 2nd generation Italian, presented an extensive slide show demonstrating his laboratory technique and the results of his IC research. I'll now try to summarize the highlights of his two hour talk with us.

1. In all the other diseases all you need to do is to identify to pathogenic (disease producing bacteria) A certain number of colonies growing within 24 hours is not required. Therefore, he believes after 50 years of experience as a micro-biologist the criteria of 100,000 colonies used by urologists is not valid.

2. If there are antibiotics in the urine, a washing procedure is necessary to see if bacteria are still present. Otherwise, bacteria will be suppressed when cultured or will appear as bizarre vegetative growth due to mutation.

3. The first morning specimen is full of contaminants and therefore the worst specimen to use for culturing.

4. 100% of IC patients have pathogenic bacteria-96.6% have either enterococcus (fecal strep) or Gaffkya- a small percentage(of which I am one) have both.

5.Broth culture medium (moist environment) is needed to grow these bacteria(agar plates won't initially work.)

6. IC is a "deep seated" infection in the bladder wall, requiring long term (3 months-1year) treatment.

7. Treatment should continue until both the culture and the esterase test(a substance released by leukocytes-a white blood cells when infection present) are negative, then continue antibiotic at least 1 month longer to treat any walled-off infection.

8. Side effects- change or decrease antibiotic. Yeast, (candida albicans) overgrowth should be treated concurrently and is not a reason for stopping antibiotic before bladder infection is completely treated.

To tell the truth, I intended to put this section of the ICD at the top, but I got to rambling, as I often do. This is the top story in this issue of the ICD, because of the rest of the story..... Strictly speaking, <Fugazotto>is not a medical doctor. He is a microbiologist, from the old school, and perhaps a bit lost in this modern age of young timber wolves.

He is an extremely nice and personable gentleman, the kind of fellow voted most likely to be someone's grandfather. Yet, he is a scrapper. <Fugazotto> is most comfortable working one on one, I gather from example. The question that has been posed I'm sure by more than one person is why don't you<Fugazotto> publish? Perhaps the answer to the maiden's prayer came on the following evening.

Quoting again from Ruth's newsletter:

The following evening, <Fugazotto> spoke with a group of urologists and other hospital personnel (IE pathologist, microbiologist etc.) at Columbia Hospital For Women, hosted by Dr. Jack B. As a result of that meeting several investigations and research projects have been initiated.

The pathologist has found bacteria (strep) in the bladder wall of a biopsy from an IC patient. The microbiologist has seen Dr. Fugazzotto's technique and is going to be attempting to grow the bacteria from a biopsy specimen.

Dr. B is planning a controlled study using antibiotics to treat IC and our support group is applying for a grant from the XXX to do a follow up study of Dr. Fugazotto's IC patients who have tried his program.

Shortly, after the meeting, a breathless Ruth called me. She gulped a time or two and said that she and her buddies were ready to make the big commitment to go for research into <Fugazotto>'s program. Boy, this takes guts! We've been disappointed so many times.

Most everything we have to work with to date is at best a cover-up. What (he) is offering is part of a real solution to the problem. Ruth and her friends have done us all a great service. They are to be commended for their foresight, and perhaps a bit of luck. What we're getting at here, is that they have some well respected MD's behind them, interested, and willing to buy into Fugazzotto's research.

No one was more surprised than Dr. B, who was just sort of fooling around after the meeting, when he found the bacteria just where said they would be. This hasn't been seen before, and confirms his assertions, at least in part.

I talked with again, after Ruth called. Sure enough, just like a complicated text book, when I picked him up again, BANG, things started to gel. The things to remember are these: The bacteria <we>are looking for are best grown in broth, au contraire' to current lab practices.

It was shown that these bacteria invade the bladder wall, hiding in and behind the normal IC scar tissue among other places, making them hard to kill. Most folks have Gaffkya, well and otherwise......

And...we came to the understanding that this is only half the problem. If indeed Gaffkya is the pathogenic cause of IC, there is the underlying physiological cause.

(The ICD believes that it is our goofy Immune System gone awry.) In other words, if most folk have Gaffkya anyway, it's the breakdown of the normal immune response, or rather that our immune response is too strong, that allows the little beasties to grow and directly damage our bladders....and our prostates, and our colons, and several female apparatuses that I ashamedly am not quite sure of.

If it could be shown that the Gaffkya organism is the agent that destroys our bladders, we would be light years ahead in our research.

This would be half the knowledge battle on the shelf right there. Personally, I find this VERY exciting. At the very least, this is the biggest news in years....and you were there!

I have made everyone's name on my mailing list available to Ruth K. I'm downright positive you don't mind. Hopefully, if the XXX sees fit, and the Virginia group continues to do well, you will receive a questionnaire in the mail at some point.

In the meantime, I need to know, and I stress this most stressfully, what your experience with<Fugazotto> 's regime has been. To show my good faith, I will start off...

I stayed on his suggested antibiotic for about a month and a half. At first, I felt better than I had for years. This lasted a couple of weeks. Everything improved, except frequency. Bladder, colon, general well being, everything but my pea-sized bladder.

After the 1st month, the program leveled off, and it looked like I was going back to my usual self, so after a little longer I stopped the medication. Like you, long term drugs bothers me, and also maybe like you, money was a little tight, and my drug of choice was darned expensive.

Normally, you can't see thru my urine specimen for the bacteria, (which never cultured..snicker), but while on the antibiotic my specimen improved dramatically. My doctor was a bit boggled by the improvement. <Fugazotto>told me in my last conversation that I could probably have cut back on medication at that point. He stresses that you have to stay on the program.

I am presently awaiting more bountiful days to get back on the program and stay on it. Everybody else I have talked to, to date, has told me about the same thing. I have not heard from a single person who says they are cured. So there! It's out now.

Let me hear from you about your success or lack of it. While I don't personally have a success story to report, I don't have a report from anyone who thinks they did the program as well as they could have either.

One thing that I did hear about was the reluctance of the treating physician to place someone on a long term antibiotic program. What can I say? We're on the leading edge with this thing. Will it pan out? I hope so. I hope so.

The IC Disclaimer Issue 8

THE IC DISCLAIMER THE BIMONTHLY NEWSLETTER FOR INTERSTITIAL CYSTITIS
YOUR EDITOR: NORMAN MORRISON
THIS MONTH: "K REPORT"

I have been following a story that is still unfolding as I write this. As you may recall from past issues, we have been looking at the work of Dr. Fugazzotto, whose address will appear a little later. His work has at the same time been exciting and enigmatic. Perhaps now, in great part due to the work of Ruth K, a super volunteer for the Virginia XXX, and her friends, we may be able to shed a little light on this subject.

On October 9th of last year, Dr. Fugazotto attended a meeting and presented a slide show to the Va. group which is located close to Washington, DC. In his 2 hour talk, he explained that current microbiological thinking (ergo. your urine specimen) requires that a certain large number of bacterial colonies be found in a 24 hour period.

He, on the other hand, feels <that isn't> all that is necessary is for the med tech to find the pathogenic (disease causing) bacteria. This sounds easy, but in practice is pretty tough, because the culprit may not be the obvious candidate in the petri dish. At this point, (I'm interjecting here) the book goes out the window and long years of experience comes into play.

Following Ruth's notes now, another point is that if antibiotics are present in the urine, a washing procedure must be used, otherwise bacterial growth will be suppressed, or will appear as a vegetative growth due to mutation.

Contrary to all that's medically holy in my experience, Dr. Fugazotto says that the first urine of the morning is full of contaminants, thus the worst possible specimen to use for culture purposes, which, as you shine the light of reason upon it holds up quite well. Says Dr. Fugazotto, 100% of IC patients have pathogenic bacteria,(exactly backwards from current textbook thinking), and that 96.6% have either enterococcus,(fecal strep) or Gaffkya, and a small percentage have both.

If you did any lab work in biology class or peeked around the corner in your doctor's office you are doubtless familiar with the fate of your urine specimen. Whether done locally or elsewhere, at some point your urine is smeared on top of an agar gel solution in a petri dish, or similar.

Should bacterial growth take place, eventually the colony will encounter areas coated with various antibiotics. If growth is checked, that particular drug is indicated for treatment. Oh, there are all sorts of other things that can be done, but the main point is that it is all done on top of agar.

Dr. Fugazotto emphatically says that for our purposes, the culture must be done in a broth culture medium. If you think about it a moment, where would you as a bladder bug rather be....in a nice warm wet broth solution, or in an agar desert? Defense rests.

Perhaps, one of Dr. Fugazotto's most controversial findings is that because of the nature of the infection, it takes from between 3 months and one year of antibiotic treatment to defeat the bugs we carry. (More on this later.)

Treatment should continue until the esterase test,(a substance produced by white blood cells present at infection sites) and cultures show negative. The main side effect of prolonged antibiotic treatment can be an overgrowth of yeast, (candida albicans) which in some of us can be treated by other methods.

The story continues...... The following evening, Dr. Fugazotto met with a group of urologists and other hospital personnel at Columbia Hospital For Women, hosted by Dr. Jack B.

Some marvelous things transpired, and should be remembered by future historians of the IC struggle. After the meeting, Dr. B, a pathologist, stirred by what he heard, went back to his lab and pulled a IC bladder biopsy specimen.

Using Dr. Fugazotto's advice he found, guess what....bacteria inside the bladder specimen. That is, inside the meat, not just crawling outside. This verified for the first time, Dr. Fugazotto's theory, that the infection we suffer lurks inside our bladder tissue, behind scar tissue, and so forth.

Dr. B had only to look as Dr. Fugazotto indicated and there it was. This is indeed a breakthrough of sorts. Of course, one observation does not make it a bona fide fact. I talked with Dr. Fugazotto shortly after hearing from Ruth with these amazing details.

Let me tell you some conclusions I came to..... First. I believe that Dr. Fugazotto has hit onto something. I think he has quite possibly nailed the pathogenic cause of IC. Secondly, I think he has identified how it works by entering our bladder tissue, in a general sort of way, and thirdly, I think he's hit on the a cure for the bacteria. Also, using his methods, most any caring professional should be able to identify and treat the infection. Now, I've said it....so there!!

However.....and there's always a big ol' however.....Dr. Fugazotto and I agreed that the bacterial infection was only half of the problem. Please listen carefully. There is every possibility that there are a great many people walking around with Gaffkya, and all the rest who may never have a urinary problem.

There has to be a reason that we, you and me, are wide open to the propagation of the bacteria. It has to do with allergies, or enzymes, or brain damage, liver warts, or a million other causes. WE JUST DON'T KNOW!

Why do we get IC and no one else? We know for a 99% fact that it isn't catching, although it may be passed from generation to generation.

Lordy, don't go get an abortion on that account. I'd have rather lived with it than not to have lived.......

The very exciting thing to remember here is that until now, even with the best of intentions, a researcher had very little in the way of facts to go on to start up a research project. Dr. Fugazotto has eliminated that excuse. We now have a very meaty proposition to sink our teeth into indeed....the pathogenic cause of IC.

And, we have the tools, staining techniques, preliminary statistical findings, growth techniques, and the rest thanks to the good doctor to get started in a big way. Of course, we have one more thing.

Dr. Fugazotto will come to your meeting to present his findings at his expense. Yes....at his expense. I will insert here, that of course, you would no doubt make it worth his while, like, a well publicized state meeting with the medical gentry in attendance or the like.

You should provide lodgings and such. Why does he do it? I talked to him for nearly an hour....Beats me all to heck. He's just one of those real nice folks you meet from time to time.

I must say in closing this part of the ICD that no one has yet called or written and stated that they have been cured using Dr. Fugazotto's technique. On the other hand, no one has called and told me that they have followed his prescription to the letter either, including myself.

Be advised that your doctor will put up a bitch, and it is dreadfully expensive, although your druggist will rave about it. Fiscal problems aside, and lack of hard research to the rear, I think that this line is our current best hope of resolving at least half of the IC mystery.

We owe it to ourselves and those to follow to further this research any way we can. Think about it..........
Thanks to Ruth K. I say it three times....thanks. Ruth and her wild Washingtonians are just about to launch into some preliminary studies of Dr. F.'s findings, also, they are charged with keeping a fire lit under Dr. B, who's planning his own study on this subject.

They are gearing even as you read this to get some statistics on the issue. She needs your input. Call her at (X). Gosh, we both had a super chat on the phone a while back. We were so excited that if she and I were in the same room, we'd probably have tossed the cat down in the floor and danced a jig around it.

The IC DISCLAIMER is non-profit, but not tax deductible. One year costs $7.00. It is published 6 times a year. Please make your check payable to: Norman Morrison, the editor of this magazette.

Back issues as available are at regular prices Write. THANKS! All correspondence is considered public unless you specify otherwise. Your address may be made available to others with similar interests unless you say otherwise. KEEP WRITING!

Well now. My favorite time. Time to do a little back-pedaling. Fact of the matter is I'm a little late with this issue. Some of my new readers anted up and *poof* where did Norman go. Well, beats me folks. My lateness at this page will not be attributed to two things....lack of time, or laziness. Call it writers block.

I've developed a lot of theories...none which I'm satisfied with. Call it a vacation. I don't know what to call it. Anyway, I appreciate your patience as I put the whole ICD operation on hold thru the holidays. We're back on track now, and as I plan to speed up the next couple of issues, you must continue to endeavor to persevere.

Maybe all this started with my Sears riding lawnmower breaking the middle of last summer. I've put everything off since then. The mower finally went to the shop yesterday. (A host of funny looks just erupted from my computer screen, just behind these words...) Oh well........

HINT If you suffer from bad bowels like yours truly, associated with IC, you may be encouraged to know that I think I've found one of life's little links. Due to my schedule, and financial status, I eat an extraordinary amount of burgers. They are relatively cheap, especially the cheap ones, and quick.

I think I have found a silly, but painful fact. You know those little sesame seed things on the buns.....I believe they contribute greatly to our sitting problems. When they hit the lower intestines, they irritate, either from a digestibility, or chemical standpoint, our little gutties.

We then have trouble sitting. Since I've laid off the seeded bun varieties I've felt much better. A real test of this is the Arby's brand goods. Their buns are covered with some real little black looking seeds. These produce a guaranteed gut wrench at sitting time.

Also, guys, before I forget, Dr. Fugazotto agrees that the bacterial infection can also reach down into the prostate, causing all sorts of problems.... Please let me know if you try the seedless regime and have success.

I surely stepped into it last ish, when I said something like..."You don't just wake up one day and 'boom' you have IC." Several folks wrote in and said that they did in fact get IC practically overnight.

We'll cover this in more depth in the letters for the next couple of issues. While we are talking thus, be advised that I am as of now going to institute a semantics change. Instead of a broad definition called Food Allergy, we will refer to certain problems as Food Sensitivity. More on this in the next issue.

Alice N. There's that name again. AJ of Wisconsin was the first to do something that I never even thought of, and she did it again, and again, and again. She has sent stamps, travelers checks, and checks above and beyond the subscription price. She really makes getting out an issue a pleasure when it comes time to go to the printers. From all of us, thanks, and thanks again! Oh yes, she's a super nice gal to talk to, too!! (Gal, in southernese is a compliment)

THE MAILBAG

Albert A. checks in from Seal Harbor, Maine. Albert says that he's 57 and has had IC for 7 years or so. From past mail, this seems about the norm for males. Speaking of Norm, I'm 34 and have been bladder-blessed since 1982. He says that he's been on Elmiron for a couple of years and it may be helping. Glad to have you aboard, and again, many thanks for not raising a ruckus about the delay in my mail.

Beverly C, the leader of the gang in Maine sends a very nice letter. Again, I sit here shamefaced, because, several folks from that little state have written I guess mainly because of Beverly. Well, here I am.

OK...enough reproachment. Tomorrow is a work day, and my employer will make up the difference. Beverly say that she's tried bladder relaxers, anti-inflammatory medicine, Pyridium, anti-depressants, Elmiron, Angiostat...(that last escapes me for the moment?!) and Doc Gillespie.

She further says that she's hung onto hydro distension, DMSO, DMSO with steroids...(a la Jan Johnson of Ms. I believe?),baking soda, clorpactin, Gillespie's diet, aspirin, antihistamine, and something called a Helmstein procedure with alcohol cytolysis.

She said she'd let us know if the Helmstein procedure worked, but since its been awhile,(9-24...hit self on nose), and I haven't heard, I reckon it also was a no-go. Gosh, most of have tried some of these things, but I'd say you get the ICD *What the Heck* award.

Frankly, as I've said in the past, some of these procedures you mentioned that I am aware of would make the sinister Dr. Mengele blush.

Sheesh. Beverly didn't hesitate to mention that she came down with IC after a 4 day child birth labor. (Editor shaking head...he has two kids.....C-section heh heh).

She says she had a fever and it came on overnight, and she knows of a couple of others who came up with IC in a similar manner. Well, one thing is for sure, we all know now that it can be sudden, and from this and other letters, all I can say is that this sure tightens up the case for it being some kind of hormonal thing. I guess I'm weird, but our second child was a very hard birth....for me. Yep....The night after the happy event, I was so depressed that I scarfed down 8 whiskey sours and never even got wobbly.

Usually, I can smell alcohol and get lopsided. I don't know why I got depressed...I wasn't unhappy. It was a deep, dark depression, the like I've never had before. It came on the day that V had C and was gone the next, but sure enough, it wasn't long after until my case of IC started coming on. Coincidence? I've always wondered about that. Also, I seem to have monthly or bi-monthly cycles of water weight gain and such. I have always suspected that my wife infected me with something.(Not Really).

But, my IC gets worse and better relatively speaking on an orbit around these cycles. Anybody else out there run into this?? Beverly says that she's in constant pain and has had IC since age 23. With one kid, a full time job and trying to take a course at a local university, she's got her hands full, and as those of us know who have IC, having IC is already a full time job.

On bad days you can get pretty worn out just trotting and hurting before you ever factor in work. Beverly says she's got a good support system. I guess most of the folks who write in do, Beverly. We are awfully lucky that way. I'm probably not as nice as the folks who have to put up with me. We have much to be thankful for.

Finally, Beverly asks how I got her name. Well, a very kind young lady sent me the eastern XXX state coordinator list. Without it, I'd be flying blind for sure. Every time the newsletter goes out, I broadscatter a half dozen freebies in the US, and some Canada.

So far, no word from Canada, but the ICD was definitely a hit in Maine. If anyone has an updated list out there, I'd sure like a copy. Also, I don't have address one from across the Mississippi.

The whole western US is off limits until I can get one of my feets into the door. If you should have a list, or even an address of a Coordinator, it just might turn the trick.

We don't get any favors from the XXX corporate here at the ICD. For the new reader, the name of this magazette was a play on words. Seemed like every other word from the home office had a disclaimer in it. Heck, the whole medical community acts like they aren't even sure there is such a thing as IC, hence the name IC Disclaimer.

I also have a disclaimer or two, but I hope and pray that common sense will always prevail out there and that you will seek out the best medical advice you can find. In the absence of medical advice on little matters like surviving with IC, however, the ICD carves out its little niche with helpful hints from all over the country from survivors.

I just re-read a nice letter from AJ. It's a bit dated now, but she mentions that she's disappointed in Oprah. Well, I'm disappointed too. I got my letter back from her and immediately filed it.

I also wrote to Doc Bob Lanier in Texas who has a syndicated minute that runs on various news shows. No go. He did do a segment on how men could best remove themselves from their trouser zippers. I guess that's kinda like IC.

Frankly, you could not pay me enough to be on Oprah, even for the cause, but I sure wish Bob would come across with a piece. (Bob is going to get his usual copy of this magazette.) I talked to her last night and she said she was writing a letter to the president. Get 'em Alice Jane!!

Beth M....your back issues as I have them are on the way. Kindly forgo the usual buck apiece charge. I just found your check in your letter, neatly stapled. Vicky (wife) just hollered at me....Screeeech!!!

Beth writes from Alexandria, Va... Boy, are some of you going to be surprised when that check you forgot all about comes in this month's batch. Well, I'm honest, if not right bright. Guess who balances the bank books around here?? (Back-peddling again)

We'll end this issue here. If you find something of interest, please write. If you need to talk, you can reach me at (X). Remember, less is better. Watch what you eat, and get off the pavement once and awhile. Smell the clean air. God bless and keep you till next time....Norman

The IC Disclaimer Issue 9

THE IC DISCLAIMER THE BIMONTHLY NEWSLETTER FOR INTERSTITIAL CYSTITIS YOUR EDITOR: NORMAN MORRISON

THIS MONTH: "CATCHING UP!" 3-2

Before I get into this month's research reports, there is something that I've said in the past that I think needs retelling for our new subscribers, and its something I believe in very strongly. Never, never think that you can't possibly make a relevant and helpful contribution to the IC dilemma just because you don't have a PH.D. tacked onto the end of your name.

I guess that if I had my druthers, I'd prefer to have a practicing urologist who likes to do research come down with an especially vile case of IC. In an imperfect world this will hardly be our luck.

Instead, we have urologists and other doctors with 101 different immediate problems that demand their attention. On the other side of the coin we have a whole flock of letterless IC'ers who haven't so much as a microscope.

The IC'ers do have one thing though; a desire to terminate their IC problem. They do the best they can with what they've got, and oft times come up with some genuinely good ideas and suggestions concerning their disease of choice. Hopefully, they then send me a report so that I can in turn deliver it to you for consideration.

I emphatically want you to know that somewhere in your personal experiences with IC may lie an important piece of the puzzle. Don't sell yourself short.

On the same line, most of you know me only through the ICD. Actually, I have a life outside of IC. A pretty good one, as a matter of fact. I was having such a good life over the holidays that I got a bit behind on the ol' ICD, to which I'm addressing some quality catch up time.

I go hunting, and fishing, work two jobs and ever so often as needed do volunteer work of one sort or the other. I'm a semi-retired Jaycee. Even though I've got plenty to keep me busy, I'm NOT a workaholic. Leave that to the Ulcerites.

I know the value of taking a break once in awhile. You too, must remember that it is OK to rest every now and again. Just having IC is a full time 24 hour job before you ever punch the time clock. Don't forget to take time for yourself once in awhile. I can wait.....but not too long...(ha ha).

The mail has been kind to me since our last chat dear friends. In the still catching up department, I've been eagerly awaiting the chance to go over Valerie Z's last correspondence. Valerie is an upstate NY girl with a hefty case of IC and a lot of research. She opens by saying that she agrees with my theory of the 4 stages of IC...You know, stage one is where you are having pressure on the bladder to stage four (end stager) like me with a thimble sized receptacle. Also, the worse your IC, the more foods your are sensitive to. She says that she knows several people who have stopped IC progression by modifying their food intake. Hurrah for them!

I just wish I had known about this earlier before mine went all the way. Read and heed, ye of moderate IC. Watch what you eat! Also, Valerie adds that dusty houses, inefficient gas appliances (like mine), perfumes, and other substances we contact daily can add to our miseries.

Car exhaust, (my 72 Nova), and printers ink can also add discomfort. I have often wondered if my burning a Coleman heater for awhile in my old tent when we would go camping for heat before going to sleep and when getting up scrambled my genes. I always did feel kind of goofy after one of those trips.

Probably just carbon monoxide poisoning, that's all. I was already brain damaged anyway....Valerie brings up an interesting point, and one that was echoed by Ruth K. Ruth doesn't know Val, and vice-versa. They both came up with this one on their own....

Hypothesis: Could the mercury amalgam that most of us have in our mouths thanks to our dentists filling our teefies be slowly dissolving, thus introducing a small but constant dose of said substance into our systems, thereby causing or aiding our IC? The proof, of course is to have all the filling yanked and replaced, or find some IC'ers without fillings. Any help out there??

OK, a follow up. Valerie went to the dentist and had a filling removed. She says,"I broke out in cysts all over my face, had a whopper of a migraine, and was dizzy and woozy for 3 days."

She said that her second trip to the dentist was much worse. I have already written Valerie on this point expressing my concern and confusion. I asked her if it could have been simply a reaction to the mouth numbies the dentist gave her. As a special treat for her visit to the dentist her IC also flared up pretty badly.

The question is, was it the drugs or the amalgam. If Valerie, and you and me, are indeed having a problem with this stuff, you can see how easily it would be to ingest a whole bait (southern for a lot) of it whilst the tooth surgeon drills and hammers happily away at the covering.

Valerie thinks she got mercury poisoning. She said that the other folks she knows who went through the same treatment did not exhibit those bad reactions. Well, what can I say? I think this idea definitely warrants further examination, since that is one thing most of us have in common. If you should decide to go this route, please let me know of your experience, and progress.

What comes next is not scientific, nor even applicable 'cept to me. Thanks for sending your last letter on that beautiful card, Valerie!

Received the other day: From my appeal for additional contacts, especially out west, I recently got a plethora of new names from an anonymous source known only to me as AGENT RAISIN. Agent Raisin would do well to check my publication (Form 007) Hiding Your Envelope Postmark before hiring out for pay. (SMILE)

Thanks from a happy Norman and standby to see what your address wreet...wrought. Finally, Agent Raisin reminds me that "We are all in this together." So we are. I invite the XXX to support and contribute to the ICD with articles and information. You have but to mention a need to this editor for the same consideration.

Melanie B, Regional XXX Coordinator sends her best. For those of you who don't know her, she watches over the South East like a mama eagle caring for her chicks. She helped me get the ICD started, and is one of the best things the XXX management has going for it. She says that she tried (Feldene?) for arthritis and got a bad IC setback.

Folks, we just never know what's going to affect us. Wherever we can, we must go slowly. With medicine, this isn't usually possible, but just the same. . . . Melanie brings up a point that is particularly relevant to me. Heredity.

We know absolutely nothing about IC and heredity. She worries that her daughter may be coming down with IC. Her docs tell her not to worry. Hers is not the first time I've seen this manifestation. How can I put this or even, should I put this issue up for a look. The worst business you can mess with is family business.

Personally, (dadgummit, I really didn't intend to get into this) I have two kids. They aren't big enough yet for me to be worrying, but still I worry. Her child is coming of IC age now, and Melanie says that she's seeing signs. I HOPE NOT. Melanie is one of the smartest IC'ers around, and if she says she see something, you'd better listen. On the other hand, I hope she's wrong. Science tells us that there is absolutely no reason to consider IC a generation to generation thing. It could skip your kids and affect theirs, or theirs, or no one. (<**Editor 2014:** Fresh anecdotal evidence. My old kids, who were little kids at the time of the ICD are now big kids in their early thirties. No sign of IC! Dittos for the grand young'uns.)

From extremely far afield, let's bring the plane in for a landing with the rest of the mail....

Let me extend a tremendous welcome to Mary R, the Upstate NY XXX Coordinator. Mary, please feel free to show your copy of the ICD around to your friends if you see something worth discussing. The ICD is not out for mail volume, just balanced coverage around the country through good folks in the know like yourself.

Of course, if one of your flock wants their own copy, well, we can handle it that way too. The ICD goes international!! Welcome Marjorie O'P from Canada. We've been looking forward to this for a long time now.

Marjorie indicates that the ICD's current obsession, Dr. Fugazotto is news to her, and be this the case, perhaps to the rest of the Canadians too. Well, standby. The lower 48 is all abuzz over the good doctor's findings on the bacterial nature of IC. The next issue of the ICD is dedicated to the whole area of modern microbiology as related to urinology.

I know you'll find some interesting stuff coming up. On the subject of Dr. Fugazotto, as many of you may already know, he just went through a pretty good heart surgery. A recent phone call to his new assistant Georgia confirmed that he is doing well, and recovering nicely. The main problem she is having is keeping restrained till his new chest equipment gets settled in.

I can imagine. I was talking with him in his room at UAB in Birmingham when the doctors came in with their suggestions on multiple bypasses. It never fazed him. When they left, he picked right up where he left off in our conversation. We'll talk at length about this in the next issue.

AJ, the ICD's unofficial silent partner writes. She asks if anyone out there ever feels like they are sitting on a can of worms? Well, as a matter of fact, I felt that way last nite after a day of trotting to the bathroom. Must have been something I 'et, as Grandpa Morrison reputed to have said one time.

I attribute the feeling to a simple and temporary case of hemorrhoid flare up, as it is called on the television ads. Does anyone else have this?

It's official now.... It's confirmed that Dr. Bob Lanier will air a segment on IC sometime in June on his syndicated TV show called, 60 SECOND HOUSECALL. His show is currently seen in 42 markets around the country.

His one minute explanations of all things medical usually air within local newscasts. He comes across as the kind of doctor we all want and occasionally find, and he delivers more good info in 55 seconds than you can get on a year's worth of the evening news with Dan, whathisname.

Score one for the ICD. With what we sent him, and what he'll dig up, I expect that a great many of the ICunawares out there will come into the fold. It's a blessing to finally find out what's been eating at your vitals after years of fruitless searching!

If you should be in an area that broadcasts Dr. Bob, you can call your local TV station in late May and ask them to tell you when the segment airs. I plan to keep a copy and later, if you want to see it we can make arrangements to let you send me a tape to record over on.

You know what? I just erased a whole page of text...again! One of these days, I vow to take a large and powerful magnet to this software. I will pass it back and forth, up and down, and generally around in a random motion and erase the darn thing, then give it to my kids to use as a square frisbee. (<**Editor 2014:** I was referring to a 5.25" floppy. No one under the age of 40 in 2014 would know what a 5.25" floppy is. Go look it up.)

Now let's see, where was I? Yes...Peggy T. Peg sends in a super letter from Pennsylvania. I was just thinking how nice it is to be making friends all over. Peggy says that her buddy, Mary LC, the Penn State XXX Coordinator showed her the last copy and she thinks it's great. You haven't seen anything yet...wait till the next issue.

Peggy is one of those girls who help keep our statistics so dismal. She says that she has had IC since 1975, but just got diagnosed last year. It's not funny at all, but still for those of us who have been there it is darkly funny that 3 separate specialists took her money only to tell her that she didn't really have a problem.

Finally, she found a urologist who not only diagnosed her problem, but told her about the XXX support group network. Verruh unusual. How many of us learned that there were others out there with IC from our doctor?

She said that oral medication left her a zomboid, so she went the ol' bladder infusion route. She said that she had 22 weeks of DMSO and DMSO with steroids. Lately, she and her (He has got to be a nice and patient fellow) husband have been pumping Sodium Cromalyn and Marcaine in the bladder via a catheter at home.

These drugs are new to the ICD. She has also added Heparin to the mix, which is by all accounts the standard. Peggy also agrees with an ICD standard. She said that for two weeks she had cause to remember in exquisite detail a delightful trip to an Italian restaurant. This, of course, begs for a question. What do Italians with IC eat?

What do Americans with IC eat, and live not to regret? Interesting line, and one the ICD is very interested in.

Finally, Peggy says that she is very interested in the work of Dr. Fugazotto. She asks what his remedy is, what types of drugs and how long. It was a bit of a job, Peg, but I think your questions will be answered in the next issue of the ICD, so stay tuned.

Peggy, in true ICD form offers her mailbox and phone number. If you would like to correspond with another member of the IC species, compare notes, and what, write Peggy at: Peggy T, Dover PA.,. Thanks Peggy, looking forward to hearing more from you.

Write. THANKS! All correspondence is considered public unless you specify otherwise. Your address may be made available to others with similar interests unless you say otherwise. KEEP WRITING!

Many references have been made to Dr. Fugazotto in this issue. For the new reader, in short, the ICD has been quite taken, as have many of its readers by the original research of this gentleman that tends to show that IC is the result of a bacterial infection which is news in the IC community. Of course, there's much more to IC than this, and we'll get into it in-depth in the next issue.

Suffice to say, though, that this is the most unique finding, in the ICD's opinion of the century in so far as our favorite malady is concerned. I want to give you something to think about between now and the next issue.

I don't know what all it takes to get a new procedure on the market. But I would guess that repetitive proof certainly helps. Each and every one of you has had multiple urine tests done. Most likely, your doctor uses a dedicated medical lab somewhere, whether in a hospital or in a remote location.

I want to ask you to think about how you could get in touch with this lab and see if their management would be willing to try and duplicate Dr. Fugazotto's findings. Again, and for the last time, we will explore this idea further in the next issue. I have been doing some work on this already, and believe it or not....it's not easy. However, this kind of thing will have to be done, and I think a grass roots effort on our part can speed it along.

As mentioned earlier, the ICD goes west of the Mississippi on a reader foray for the first time this issue. For purposes of trivia, I might mention that we pretty well have the east coast covered, all the way up into Canada. We go where it always and never snows. (No pun intended.) I hope our friends out west find something of worth in this little magazette and will spread it around a bit.

Many generous thanks to Ruth K and the fired up Virginia gang for their pioneering work into proving out Dr. Fugazotto's work. One other note from their super newsletter, a local member reports that if you are taking Norflox, you must stay away from antacids. Like the Va. newsletter, all correspondence means life or death to the ICD.

If you have a newsletter, please put me on the list, and otherwise, keep those letters coming. Remember to print all names of medicines and medical terms you report on. I won't be able to attend the XXX conference in May due to my financial situation....I believe this is the disclaimer most folks use. I had planned to leave it at this, but after reading Mary R's (Upstate NY Coordinator) excellent newsletter, I came upon a realization that I'd like to share.

I know that several of my readers will be going to New Orleans in May, and all would like to. Of course, I hope that those who are able to attend will send the ICD a report and any info they come upon that they feel like the rest of us may profit by.

I'm counting on your generosity in this area. (Be sure to say hello to Dr. Fugazotto on my behalf.) The point I'd like to make is that like Mary, many, I'm sure, who will attend will do so with some personal financial discomfort. The fact is that some who go will come back to face several meals of Vienna sausages because they had to spend the cookie money to get there.

AND, whether you fly or drive, traveling with IC is always an adventure. We appreciate your sacrifice. If you should be traveling on I-20 between Bham and Atlanta on the way down, be sure to holler. (Phone number). I'll be glad to give you a tour of the ICD building...(my dining room) and offer cocktails... (Sprite in a can.) We have also recently moved the bathroom into the house! How about that.

The best way to help yourself is to watch what you eat. We have all sorts of hints and tips by and by in the ICD, but in the meantime, just remember what you eat can hurt you three days later. Use a little common sense, because while we can't yet cure IC, most of us can at least manage it. We may not manage it to our satisfaction, but for many, any relief at all is a Godsend.

Till next issue, take care, watch what you eat, and write! God Bless. Norman

The IC Disclaimer Issue 10

THE IC DISCLAIMER

    THE BIMONTHLY NEWSLETTER FOR INTERSTITIAL CYSTITIS

    YOUR EDITOR: NORMAN MORRISON

    THIS MONTH: "URINARY SAMPLING TECHNIQUES

    (A very important issue indeed! Editor)

I had a devil of a time coming up with an acceptable name for this month's issue. Most folks, as you know go eeeee-yuk at the thought of a little stray urine. Like I say, if urine scares you, you'd better contract some other syndrome besides good ol' IC.

This month we'll explore two issues that should be of current interest. First, we'll take a look at a modern multi-function medical lab and secondly we'll take <a look> at Dr. Fugazoto's unique techniques as explained to me by the man himself.

On March 2nd of this year I had the distinct pleasure and honor to tour the medical laboratory facilities of the (<city name> regional hospital facility in Northeast Alabama. Editor).

I found the staff to be supportive and genuinely interested in my tales of IC. Among the nice folks I talked with, let me mention these names: Janice M, Betty J, Delores K, Larry H, Alex O, and Bill T. I fairly glowed as I walked out into the rainy morning following the tour.

Although I saw many interesting things, I will confine my comments mainly to bacterial culturing of urine samples.

Have you ever wondered what happens to your 2 ounces or so when the nurse disappears down the hall?

Larry H, Supervisor of Microbiology gives us these facts: Generally, a clean catch, that is, a regular sample....(not employing a catheter or the like) is placed in a test tube containing a stabilizing compound. Said compound inhibits growth of the possible bacterial components, regulating them. They are then logged in.

Next, we grab a petri dish, (remember, from school, a round glass dish with a lid) containing either agar, (pronounced ah-ger) with 5% sheep blood, or McConkey Agar for use in testing for Gram-Negative bacterial growth.

Let me throw this in at this point. (The Facility) routinely checks around 400-500 samples a month and only 20-30% show positive for urinary tract infection. Now, we uncork the bottle, so to speak and take a sterile, calibrated plastic loop and insert it carefully into the bottle. The tiny loop at the end of the probe (envision a tiny soap bubble maker) is retracted with precisely 1/1000th of a cc of urine.

Plop the urine down onto the agar and smear it around with a freshly sterilized wire. Place the lid onto the dish and store in an incubator. I'll bet you can guess the temperature. Yep, body temp.

After 24 hours, the sample should be showing some growth, and at 48, its time to investigate.

Assuming we've been lucky enough to catch a microbe in action, we'll find little colonies growing on the tracks we made with the sterile wire. They look much like tiny pinhead sized patches of mold growing on the red agar surface.

Remember, we deposited 1/1000th of a cc of specimen on the medium. We can count the colonies. If we find, say 50 colonies, we multiply 50 times 1000 to come up with 50,000 micro-organisms per cc. This is important. Many labs say that a person has infection only if they find 100,000 per cc.

(The Facility) advises further study when the count reaches 10,000 per cc. Keep in mind that even a healthy person may have some starving bugs floating around in their urine, so some sort of standard has to be set to determine whether or not to proceed with medication. No use in treating a healthy person with powerful and costly antibiotics.

Perhaps you remember in an earlier edition of the ICD that I referred to a method of allowing bacterial colonies to grow outward to antibiotically medicated disks. Where growth stops, treatment with that specific kind of drug is indicated. Well, that's still being done, but (The Facility) has a more precise method.

Once it is determined that further study is needed, a bit of the bacteria is scraped from the Petri dish and placed in a test tube with plain sterile water. Next, we place small drops of the resultant solution onto a MIC, or Minimum Inhibitory Concentration tray, for short. This is a clear tray, with dozens of little catch pockets.

The upper pockets are treated and will react to various kinds of bacteria, hopefully, showing the precise culprit. The lower pockets are treated with various levels of antibiotic. By seeing where growth stops, a precise dosage of said antibiotic is indicated.

Larry held an inoculated tray up to the light, and you could see, down in the bottom, a cloudy turbidity in various pockets, and none in others. The tray is put in a souped up photometer, a device that shines a light through the pockets. The intensity of the light coming through the various pockets is measured electronically, giving a precise, if roundabout, measure of growth, and consequently, after a bit of internal computation, medication dosage prescription.

Did you see me mention a microscope anywhere in the above article? Well, I didn't. The reason they don't have to rely on the light microscope is because they have a quantified, proven, system. After millions of uses, the prediction of bacterial organisms comes down to tried and true methods, practiced by trained individuals using computers. Larry's photometer incorporates a devilishly simple idea which produces super accurate results.

That, ladies and gentlemen is how we find out if and what we have in our urine. Although, my primary mission was to explore the intricacies of urine culturing, per se, I also got to examine another facet of urinalysis, which is the exploration of the components of urine. Delores K and Peggy S indoctrinated me, as best as they could into the mysteries, although, Peggy's explanations were a bit more technical that I could readily assimilate.

(She had an answer for this. Later) Employing a little machine called a Behring Rapimat, Delores treats little chemstrips with urine and runs them through. A short time later, the instrument produces a little printout with a lot of vital info.

Like me, I'm sure you are familiar with some of the stuff, and not with others. We find the levels of Leukocytes, (white blood cells....amazing!), Nitrite, PH balance, Protein, Glucose, Ketones, Bilirubin, Blood, Urobilonogen, and Ascorbic Acid.

At a glance, obviously, a great many things about the health of the patient can be seen, since the normal levels, (Keeping in mind that other variables such as age, weight, lifestyle, and medical problems, etc.) must be taken into consideration. It is much to my disgrace that I did not take a tape recorder with me to talk to these two ladies.

As I told them, everyone in IC circles says that it may be caused by (Get out the band....) some component of urine, but no one is doing anything to prove it. Perhaps she will allow me to come back sometime to get information in this area to do a special report in a future ICD. I have no shame.

Oh yes, finally, a microscope. Delores can tell a lot of things by what her trained eye spots under the lens. And finally, Peggy recommends that anyone, (actually, she was talking to me, hmmmnnn) who is interested in these topics should try to reference books by Todd and Sanford, or Davidson and Henry.

Also, a nifty way to see what's been found recently can be had by checking out Leukocytes and related topics in the magazine section. This topic should be broad enough to bring a lot of the aforementioned areas into play. In summation of this segment, I would just like to say once again, and especially now that I have seen the incredible technology available to us, certainly, if we could but find some interested researcher somewhere, with access to this equipment, funding, and a mission, many of our toughest questions should prove answerable.

In the meantime, Peggy says that a quick course or two at a local college couldn't hurt. An hour or two spent with one of my co-workers college books on Microbiology confirms that for me, and I'll bet you, getting smarter and a good grade to boot shouldn't be too difficult, assuming you can find the time.

Many thanks to all the nice people at (The Facility) for helping me to fortify my foundation in the study of what's been hurting me.

<Fugazotto>

Several years ago, a doctor came down with a mysterious ailment. He was in so much pain, and had to urinate so frequently that he had to close down his office. After much searching for an answer to his unusual problem he finally contacted a gentleman by the name of Paul Fugazotto who at that time was in charge of the Nevada State Health Laboratory.

Fugazotto, a microbiologist by trade, set about to find the answer. The accepted techniques of the day, (still used today) provided no answers. He reasoned that his patient was evidently in trouble, and where there's smoke, you'll find fire.

The key, Fugazotto felt, lay in the nature of the problem. He had a pathogen which thrives in a decidedly wet urinary environment and one which was not detectable by ordinary means. Standardized tests were of no use. Employing non-standard urinary techniques, he did indeed discover the cause of the doctor's problem and in time after taking the right antibiotics did become much better.

When your urine specimen goes to Dr. Fugazotto, it is grown out on a Petri dish in the standard way as a check, but then the method takes a sharp turn. Without going into detail, I'll tell you the main difference between his method and that of the standard lab.

First, your urine is washed in a sterile solution to remove all growth inhibitors such as synthetic antibiotics and even naturally occurring suppressants made in your own personal chem-lab, your body.

Next, and most importantly, a culture is obtained using a liquid broth medium instead of agar.(He also employs the standard agar method as a control.)

Dr. Fugazotto has found that the pathogen he has come to recognize, namely Gaffkya just won't perform on the standard agar plate. Lastly, when the incubation period has been satisfied he looks for the bacterial pathogens which he recognizes with the help of a microscope. He is only interested in finding these specific little bugs. The other common opportunistic bacteria such as e.Coli are ignored.

If you remember, in the standard test, the lab tech is looking for 10 to 100 thousand organisms per cc. Dr. Fugazotto is only interested in finding what he considers to be the specific pathogen, Gaffkya.

Enterococcus is also common. If he finds them, he's nailed his bug and the source of our problem. He says that 99% of all people who have IC also have these pathogens lurking in their urinary tract. Dr. Fugazotto agrees that it is quite likely that these little critters can also find a home in our prostate glands, should we have one, and in our intestines. The main way that his technique and that of your neighborhood med lab differs is that he uses a broth solution to grow his cultures, and in his opinion, if any of his target bacteria are found, it's a darn good indicator that plenty more are present.

He is looking for the pathogen, not an x amount, as in regular procedures. In the area of treatment, Dr. Fugazotto diverges from the norm too. Most often he'll recommend a specific antibiotic, which is normal enough, but then advises that treatment proceed for 3 months to a year. The Gaffkya infection is deep seated and near-impossible to wipe out, so long term treatment is indicated. As you know, most antibiotic courses lasts only a week or two.

This gives medical men and patients alike a moment of pause. All I can say is that I know of several folks who are using his method, and aside from the sometimes inevitable irritation caused by any medication I haven't had any bad reports. Any time you are on long range medication you should make sure to have your various fluids monitored by your doc to make insure all is well.

Our challenge is to get Dr. Fugazotto's methods standardized. If you may recall, Dr. Fugazotto is recovering from some splendid heart surgery, but he does indeed have a helper by the name of Georgia, with whom I've had a couple of nice conversations. I would like to do on paper what I've done on the phone and say, "Thanks, Georgia." Nice name, too.

The IC DISCLAIMER is non-profit, but not tax deductible. One year costs $7.00. It is published 6 times a year.

You can help speed the standardization of Dr. Fugazotto's research along a bit. Somewhere, locally, or far off, there is a medical laboratory that does your fancy urinalysis. You can find out who they are through your doctor.

If you would like to help, contact them and tell them a bit about Dr. Fugazotto's unique approach to culturing urine samples and ask if they might be able to find the time to help and verify his results. If you click, you can either contact the good doctor or me. Either way, it is my understanding at this time that they will receive a description of the procedure and whatever other data Dr. Fugazotto feels would help them.

This is an area that you could make an immediate and valuable contribution. You never know until you ask. Now, before we all jump up and down hurrahing, there's one little problem.

We still have a little problem. As good as Dr. Fugazotto's approach is, it's still like trying to come in through the back door. There's a good chance that a lot of well people are walking around with the same organisms in their system that we have, yet ours go on to feast on our innards and theirs don't. Chances are that the root of the problem lies in a mis-behaving immune system. If we could lick that problem, I believe the pathogenic side of IC would take care of itself.

While Dr. Fugazotto's research has given us a definite foothold in the bacteria department, we still have our immune thing to contend with. This doesn't diminish the importance of pathogenic IC in any way. It just keeps it in perspective. At least, while I see little to no movement in the immune area, Dr. Fugazotto has made the discovery of the century as far as our condition is concerned. At least that's the way I read it. How about you?

By the way, I'm into my second week of Dr. Fugazotto's recommended antibiotic treatment and all is going fine. I am, of course, feeling a lot better.

Got another one for you....From Kay R, Alabama's Assistant XXX Coordinator comes word of an antihistamine called Trinalin. Its Norm Tested, a report to follow...

I chanced to talk to Kay a while back and she told me that she has allergy trouble, amongst other things with dust. Well, I do too. This funky winter and super early spring has played the devil with my IC. You know, it seems like whatever you are already sensitive to gets ten times worse.

Kay told me that she has had IC for a long time and quite by chance she found that Trinalin helped her IC. I told her that I doubt it would help me, because I can't even safely take an aspirin.

She agreed and said she was in the same boat, but just the same, the stuff works. Seems like a year or so ago, her doctor prescribed it for the sniffles, and she found that it tremendously improved her IC. What the heck, I got some and tried it. She takes two a day, but me, being a cautious type take them only when I really need them.

To make a long story short, the first time I popped one, I got a huge case of acid tummy. I nearly banished them forthwith, but, being from Guinea, my inquisitive nature took over and I swallowed another one a couple of days later. I've never had the acid problem again. The stuff seems to indeed help the pain, and it has definitely moderated a most pollenful spring.

I have found that it works best when taken at bed time. It helps you to rest because it makes you a wee bit drowsy. By the morning, the drowsies have worn off but the good part keeps working most of the day. If you have a problem with pollen and dust, you might consider giving it a shot. Like I say, I take it as needed. Kay takes the full daily dosage which is two. Whatever floats the boat.

If you try it, you are required by the ICD to let me know how it works...thumbs up or thumbs down. Also, should you try this or any medicine, herb tea, goats milk, whatever, and see that it's hurting your bladder...quit. What works for one may really mess someone else up. Be careful. If you think white chocolate is safe to eat for instance,....well....

Speaking of dust....You can write for some free material on allergies from the American College of Allergy and Immunology, <Address defunct>. They will send you information on several different things and the addresses of all board certified allergists in your area.

Included is a tract on the house dust mite. These little critters live in your bed and eat your dead skin. If that isn't bad enough, they die and blow up your nose, complicating your already complicated allergy situation. Gad! Just when you thought it was safe to turn out the light!

I think I can say with this issue, the ICD is caught up.

Looking back through the mail, I find a letter from Linda R, a member of the Alabama gang in Birmingham. Linda wrote me some time ago and asked where in the heck was the ICD. I wrote and told her I had went hunting for the first time in 5 years. Some of your checks waited for an embarrassing length of time before getting cashed. Guess what. I think I forgot to cash Linda's. It goes back to October. Just goes to show you that IC affects men's brains as well as bladders.

Linda had mentioned that most medicines make her feel worse and only on the best of the good days will she toss a coke. Is it not amazing how a little pain will make you lose interest in your former favorite foods?

She says that in Birmingham some women are opting, (were opting? How is it coming?) for the Infusaid Implantable Infusion Pump which puts medication right on the spot. Unfortunately, she says that she has one sister who is diagnosed with IC and another with bladder problems. I don't know what this means. Is it heredity?

Could it be something common in the environment where they were raised? I said last issue that Melanie B was concerned about her daughter. Linda too, says that she hopes it's not something that must be passed on. Finally, Linda mentions our good friend way down in Mississippi, Jan J. Jan ties quite a few folks around the country together. Haven't heard from her in awhile.....hint.... I hope Linda (you) let us know how the infusion pump thing is working out.

Sometimes, doing the ICD is like looking at a big darkened map of the United States with little glowing lights where you live. All of a sudden, POOM, one really lights up. Such a one is Ruth K and her fired up Va. folks.

Most of you know that they have been funded by the XXX to carry on research into the results of Dr. Fugazotto's work. We wish you all much success and God speed. In her newsletter, she also says a local allergist has found enterococcus in semen samples of men who are married to IC gals. I infer that the reverse could also be true. Perhaps we should give some thoughts to getting a bit of treatment for our partners, should we eventually find out that Gaffkya and enterococcus can be transmitted back and forth like a yeast infection.

Keep in mind that a healthy individual without the IC immune problem has little to nothing to fear from these little buggers, but could possibly serve as a carrier. Something to think about. What do you think? Again, I thank you for your newsletters, letters and general support.

Since this issue was written before our way out west campaign results are known, I'll tell you how we fared in our subscription campaign west of Jan J.

Till next issue, keep writing, and God Bless. Norman Oh, one last thought....always one of those lately.

Seems like that I was in the hospital the other day for a 2 year 24,000 gallon checkup of my plumbing. Thankfully, the doctor found that my bladder was as crummy as ever. He said he was going to stretch it a bit, but as usual chickened out when he saw what a sorry state it is in......Well, anyway, nothing new to report....that's the main thing. Checkup OK.

While I was interned, I had the opportunity to look around a bit, and I wanted to tell you, that as poor, pitiful as we with IC are.....ladies and gentlemen, there are many and worse things out there. Let us always be thankful for what dignity we do have left. Let us also remember that many folks out there don't enjoy the support net we do. Things can always be worse. A short visit to the hospital can be good medicine. Take care....Your friend...Norman

The IC Disclaimer Issue 11

THE IC DISCLAIMER THE BIMONTHLY NEWSLETTER FOR INTERSTITIAL CYSTITIS
YOUR EDITOR: NORMAN MORRISON
THIS MONTH: "THE 7% SOLUTION

A big welcome to all the new readers we seem to have fetched since the last issue. You know something? This issue has the feel of starting all over again, in a way. Seems like I was about to bust wide open to divulge what I had learned in that opener, and it is so now.

I've started this ICD over and over in my mind....so many times, in fact, that the way it looks now is exactly backwards from what I had in mind all along.

And another thing. I've been in the know for a month or so, and have resisted temptation to just blabber like a complete and joyful idiot, which is close to the way I am anyway. I've seen naught to change my mind, so here goes.....in a minute.

First, I must take a moment to recognize two people who help to make the ICD possible, and a third who has been at the center of the news. Since I'm going backwards, I'll mention Ruth K first. You have seen that name several times over the last two or three issues. I was talking to my wife the other night about Ruth, when I said, "What would we do without Ruth?"

After I had said it, I told Vicky that I believed I would put that statement of fact into the next ICD.

Q.E.D. At the present time Ruth and her able Virginia gang are the best thing we have going for us in the IC research field; possibly the best thing we have ever had going for us in the last 100 years, as you shall see.

Next, I would like to mention another comer in the ICD organization. My wife, Vicky, who has always been the CEO, started as a lowly mail room clerk, (which she still is.) She has just recently been promoted to Correspondence Coordinator. She bought me a file box for my birthday and has graciously accepted the job of filing past mail. Your musings are safer than ever, dear readers!

(Editor note<2014>: I am happy to tell anyone who will listen that I'm the luckiest guy I know. The reason is because whatever else happens, I have my wife Vicky. Among other things, she cheerfully puts up with my IC, my numerous damn fool projects including book writing, and is just an all around good Christian person. Most any other woman would have booted me out the door long ago. So come what may, as long as I have Vicky, I'm the happiest and most blessed IC'er you ever saw!)

Lastly, I must tell you that in the publishing game, there are always what we call uh-ohs and things we never figured on like unpaid sample issues, word processor updates, letters to everywhere and the like. When you are on a budget, well, would be on a budget if you had sufficient capital to actually have a budget, a little monetary overage never hurts.

In this department, my good friend AJ from Wisconsin comes in mighty handy! AJ has been sending in some extra checks purt near since day one. Truly, AJ is a corner stone of the success of the ICD. Her generosity has let me have a bit of freedom mostly in correspondence that I didn't even think about when I started the ICD. She's always sending in a check or stamps, a good word, everything that's good for the garden. If we were all gathered together at this moment, I would ask you all to stand up and give her a big round of applause. I'm afraid that this little metaphysical meeting is about the best we can do right now, but it's from the heart.

The very envelopes with the ICD imprint you receive came directly from AJ's support. If any of you might wish to say hi sometime, call her at xxxx. Also, many and lush thanks to each and every Coordinator who has made mention of the ICD in their local newsletters. Heck, everybody likes to see their name in print!

Last issue was devoted to catching up on all the news. Issue 3-2 (**Editor note<2014>:** In this version it is Chapter/Issue 10) is already mostly out of print due to the fact that nearly 15 freebies were sent out west to this one and that one. I can safely report that my "WAY OUT WEST" campaign was a total bomb.

I guess that either they weren't interested, are waiting for the next free issue, or, know a bunko outfit when they see one. It's not like I was offering to sell them a lake front estate down here on Choccolocco creek or something. Oh well.

The ICD pretty well has the eastern half of the U.S. sewed up, but getting across <the> mighty Mississippi is getting to be quite a chore. Again, I ask that if you know of someone out west that might like to receive the ICD, have them contact me, or give me their address. Frankly, the new information we have coming in is just too important to keep to ourselves. Hey, don't wait on someone else to come across. There ain't no THEY, folks, it's just US.

Speaking of writing....It seems like we really got something to sink our teefies into and the mail dries up. I don't believe I've gotten any mail regarding the last two issues from any of my regulars. Surely you aren't becoming jaded by the imminent prospect of solving our little problem are you? At any one time, I would expect that I might hear from only, 20% of the readership, because everybody else is up to their eyeballs in work or something, but, this time, the lack of mail is a bit confusing. Even the threat of having to put up with me for a solid issue didn't seem to move folks to write. Hmm.

Well, never fear...the new guys have come to the rescue. We'll explore the mail a little later. The avowed goal of the ICD has been to present the latest tips and hints from our readers on surviving with IC until the magic bullet can be found. I don't intend to change that modus operandi, however, in the last year, some remarkable things have been happening out there.

Lately, I've been giving more and more coverage to the latest scientific developments. I'm afraid that at least for the next couple of issues, this will take precedence. It's for a good cause, however, as I am sure you will agree.

I haven't been too impressed with some of the more artistic efforts to define IC that have been carried on for the last few years here in the U.S. Boy, a visitor from space could readily see that a good deal of the research going on was so far out in left field that if it ever bore fruit, the eating would be ten years down the road. I couldn't even see any practical benefit from this stuff that might conceivably compliment other research, past or future. So why do it. Why support it?

Strong comments you say? Well, somebody has to say, "Whoa up there Bucky. I believe you're barking up the wrong tree."

Course, that doesn't mean anybody will listen. I spoke my mind with the ICD and a bit of down home practical advice. I mean, it's got to be pretty bad when we don't even believe in it. You old timers know how hard it was to get anybody to believe that you really had something wrong with you much less this IC stuff.

Even today...My wife was recently in the local Women's Clinic, so naturally I put her up to leaving a copy of the ICD. The gynecologist, highly trained, professionally motivated, told her that he would give the tract his personal attention....although he had never heard of this stuff called interstitial cystitis. I guess he's been in town at least 15 years.

What would you say, if I told you that I see the light at the end of the tunnel?? When I started the ICD, I never thought I'd live to make that little remark. Even as you read that, I could see that several of you raised your force shields. It even sounds a little bit like heresy to me. I can't go into detail until the next issue, principally due to the fact that the most important documents since the Ten Commandments were inadvertently chucked into the trash can by someone within my household.

Of course, since I have three variables to work with, the scientific proof of just exactly who did the deed will never come to light. However, I had 'em, and will have them again by the next issue. I can, now, however give you an overview as to just exactly what's going on. You should compliment me for being so patient, and not blabbering.

Actually, if I could talk to you face to face instead of on this paper medium, I would tend to blabber and sermonize, my voice rising, arms outstretched, etc.....

One year ago or so, we found out about Dr. Fugazotto. He held that IC is caused by a bacterial infection. Period.

He said that the bacteria were extremely difficult to culture, thus, IC folks supposedly have sterile urine. He found a way to culture these organisms. Further, he developed a treatment regimen based on long term antibiotic treatment with specifics, as indicated by his culture. I first found out about him from Melanie B, the Southeast Regional Coordinator for the XXX, and duly, if somewhat skeptically reported to you.

The next thing that happened on our road to discovery was that he attended a meeting with the Virginia IC'ers, (a-la Ruth K) where he speculated that bacteria would be found clinging to and inside of our interstitial tissue. The import of this is that if these critters prefer our meaty parts and don't fall off into the urine readily, it just gums up the discovery process all the more, hence back to the sterile urine thing.

Well, he met with Dr. B, a pathologist while he was there. B retrieved a prepared slide with tissue from some person who had suffered with IC, and sure enough, he saw bacteria right there in the interstitials. As far as we knew at the time, this was the first time this had ever been recognized by a human being...and with a regular, garden variety light microscope.

Most anybody can readily recognize that at this point we have a pretty good case for a bacterial origin for IC. (KEEP IN MIND AT ALL TIMES THAT IT AIN'T PROVEN UNTIL ITS PROVEN!)

The ICD begs for mail from folks who have been through Dr. Fugazotto's program. To this day, response has been light, but what information that has come in has pretty well shown that most everybody has had some measure of success. A theory develops. Could our autoimmune problem open us up to a bacterial infection? At this point, an excruciating game develops. Find folks who are capable and willing to duplicate Dr. Fugazotto's method of identification and treatment. I think, that to some extent this has been accomplished.

I have two hospital clinicians who are interested as well as a major drug lab. Dr. Fugazotto says that just as soon as his process is legally protected he will open it up for study by these folks.

As you know, Dr. F. is recovering from a major triple bypass surgery, and this has surely slowed things up. I have just found out that his assistant Georgia has left his employ, so I guess this puts him back to square one. Boy, this thing is beginning to read like Twin Peaks.

This brings us up to about a month ago, my time.(Mid June 1990.) Your time depends on when I get this darn thing printed and delivered! I have promised several folks who have written me a bombshell. Well here it is: Last month, I received in the mail 3 or 4 articles from Ruth K.

Judy M, one of Ruth's colleagues in the Washington DC area dug around in one of those gee whiz big libraries they have up there and came across articles from a couple of British journals including The Lancet. Three researchers over there in jolly England who have been doing work into bladder problems dating back to 1984, as far back as 1984 photographed bacteria inhabiting the bladder wall and interstitial layers in people who supposedly had sterile urine.

Using electron microspy techniques, the Brits found the cause of some if not all IC. You'd think that SOMEONE would have known that. As usual, someone else was coming to similar conclusions somewhere else, (Dr. Fugazotto.)

What we have here, ladies and gentlemen is two lines of proof of the bacterial nature of IC from two independent sources. As I said before, I am not prepared in this issue to go into the technical aspects of this work in this issue, but rest assured we will in the next. Let me continue to bring us to the present... When the delivery of these documents came, I glanced through one of the articles hurriedly, and put them down for a week or so. To be honest, I kinda flipped out a bit. I was not prepared for this.

I was and you are possibly witnessing the beginning of the end of IC. These facts that are placed on the table before you pretty much just jams the work of the last 100 years right down the toilet. If you've noticed, even on paper I've started to develop a blabbery style. To date, Ruth K and gang have approached an infectious disease specialist who intends to work on the problem, possibly delivering medicine intravenously.

I have contacted the British researchers, and am awaiting word from them. Dr. Lee N with the NIDDK (NIH) has been contacted and is very interested in exploring these new developments. We are still in expectations that Dr. Fugazotto will turn his work loose, so that we will have something to talk to the British about.

It is interesting to note briefly in this issue that the British are culturing urine samples under a 7% atmosphere of carbon dioxide, hence the name for this issue. This is their method to get the little buggers to grow. It looks like Dr. F. is far ahead of them in this area. Ruth and gang are just about to unleash the 1st ever statistical study of Dr. F.'s results. Many of you have gotten mail on this from Ruth. If you have tried the Dr. F. plan, and have not heard from Ruth and her Nova Study, by all means write to her today and get on the list to receive a questionnaire. I can't emphasize strongly enough how important this can be to us down the road.

The address is: <Address>..... It is worthwhile to note that Ruth, Judy, and friends doing this work....gosh, I don't have the whole picture, so I don't know everybody else, are doing this for flippin' free. Strictly volunteer.

They have secured a grant from the XXX to cover their major expenses. If their unpaid work of love pays off you know who will stand to profit by it aside from us; your doctor, hospital, insurance company, drug company.

It sure would be nice to get these people into the kitchen whilst the cake is being baked! Of course, and the ICD would lose too, cause you wouldn't need us any more. I reckon that'll be awhile yet, though. O.K. You tell me if I'm headed for a derailment, or have we got something here. I'll be watching the mail box.

Oh sure, there are a million and one things left to figure on. Are there more causes than bacterial for IC? Which comes first, the autoimmune problem or the bacterial problem. As Ruth and I are cautiously beginning to think it is possible that the bacterial infection is the culprit playing hob with our immune system.

How about the pregnancy connection? A lot of folks come down with IC about this time. Catheterization. Can this medical procedure damage the bladder opening it up to infection? Is it as simple as a spreading infection, as it now looks? Ruth thinks there's a chance, and good a one that it's sexually transmissible. (I would think this would only be relevant to a partner with a damaged bladder, but could pose a problem to someone with IC who after ridding herself of the infection is re-infected by the partner).

How about treatment. Standard methods may or may not work, but at the least take a great deal of time. The problem seems to be getting the medicine to the infection. The little buggers are protected by your very tissue. As the antibiotic leaches out into the urine and washes your innards, the little critters are snug behind your cells. Could intravenous treatment be the answer. Do we have the drug specifics to do the job at this time?

In men, the Brits agree with me and Fugazotto that the prostate can and does become involved. Are our colons involved also. Directly? In some roundabout way? I think it...no, I know its very likely, but which?

We have lots and lots of work to do, but the main thing is now we have a path to follow. I think. What do you think?

In the next ICD we will delve deeply into the work of these intrepid scholars from across the briny Atlantic and find out just exactly what they have to say that sets Normie on FIRE.

The IC DISCLAIMER is non-profit, but not tax deductible. One year costs $7.00. It is published 6 times a year. Write. THANKS! All correspondence is considered public unless you specify otherwise. Your address may be made available to others with similar interests unless you say otherwise. KEEP WRITING!

THE MAIL

Most all of the mail this month is from the new guys. While I was writing this edition a little while ago, the mail ran and new subscriber, Cindy L-A, the Maryland XXX Coordinator reported in. She sent a really souped up newsletter which looks like it was done on a Macintosh with a 24 pin printer, which is to say that I think everybody's newsletter looks better than mine.

I wish you could see it, but don't fret, I intend to give it a good going over in a future ICD because she has some really nice info to pass on about the physiology of the bladder, and the substance Clorpactin, a bladder wash, that sometimes does some good but no one knows exactly why type of deals. Glad to have you Cindy!

I might mention that several of the new guys have specifically requested the last issue on urine culturing. I had fun doing it, and I hope it sheds some light.

Ada P from Canton, Ga. writes. She says she has had mail from here and there, Melanie B in particular and doesn't know where in the world everybody got her address, but says she enjoys it.

Ada, I hope this issue brings you some comfort that—somebody—out there is doing some real work on our problem. May I take this opportunity to personally thank Judith M. from Va. as previously mentioned, for finding that on shelf technology I wrote of in an earlier issue. I'd say she just found our missing link, that's all. More on YOU as it develops.

*****Person Alert!!****** Does anyone out there have the address or phone number for Jan M? She called me a couple of months ago, and I must have bungled her address because I got her letter back marked wrong address. I sure would like to make good on our phone call. I have her in Milwaukee. Heck, it might be Maine. Does anyone know?

Judy M did write a very nice letter the other day. She included a bibliography of the scientific articles I've been chattering about. I will present them in the next issue. She also chided me most severely because of a slight mistake in gender I made in reference to the articles in a letter to her.....

"The British Boys as you call them are girls." O.K. So paid researchers can be girls too. There.

Received as of last week a very nice,(all the letters I get are unfailingly upbeat!) letter from Yvonne R who's over-summering in Phoenix with her daughter. At the least, she ought to get a tan. Yvonne has had IC for 4.5 years and says Dr. F.'s treatment has helped her from 3 to 10 oz. on a trip. She says she's not cured though.

Yvonne, I hope you will use some of your time out there to try and make contact with some of those western IC'ers. Welcome aboard!

Got a letter from Marjorie from Canada. I will save most of the comments for the next issue, because she really has some good comments about most everything we have discussed in the last couple of issues, and goes right to the heart of our worries and concerns about long term antibiotic usage. She mentions at the end of her letter that there is no longer a head office for <XXX?> in Canada. I certainly hope this is temporary. She says that all business has to go direct to NYork.

For my part, it has been real tough breaking into that country. Marjorie was worth waiting on, though. Marjorie mentions replacement of good bowel bugs when on extended antibiotics.

Ruth K suggests checking out Jarro-Dophilus brand whatever from your local herb shop or druggist. It replaces the good bugs that inhabit our guts. I might insert that after reading that, Ruth, I kinda wondered just exactly what kind of culture medium they use...or do I really want to know?

Welcome to Barbara McKs from Canastota New York. Looking forward to getting a shaggy letter from you on what's doing. Well, that about closes out this issue. Look for some in-depth analysis of the British Girls findings, a little soul searching with Marjorie O'P's points. I've been doing it ever since I declared for Dr. Fugazotto's research, so jump in, and whatever else the mail brings. Take care, watch what you eat, and God bless.

The IC Disclaimer Issue 12

THE IC DISCLAIMER THE BIMONTHLY NEWSLETTER FOR INTERSTITIAL CYSTITIS
YOUR EDITOR: NORMAN MORRISON
THIS MONTH: "WE WRAP UP BACTERIA"

On behalf of the rest of the ICD gang, I would like to especially welcome our new crop of readers since last issue. For the older folks, know that we have indeed broke the Mississippi barrier. We are out west now. We are just getting started in the west but word of mouth is a wonderful thing.

A sad note for my part... I want to tell everybody that has written lately that the reason I haven't responded personally this time around is that 5 weeks ago my very active 75 year old father had a big stroke. Vicky and I are both only children and we have been put in a position of a man standing between the swamp and a hungry alligator.

My mom has moved in with us, the business that my father and I were in is in retched shape, but must be maintained at least for the next few months by yours truly alone, along with my other job etc. We just placed him in a nursing home yesterday. He is in a facility that is 70 miles away, and the bills are just starting to come in. Any of you that have had to face this know what's happening just now.

I had tried to prepare myself for father's demise, but this has really knocked me for a loop. This wasn't in the plans. The good news is that he's in a Veterans home...the only one of its kind in the nation, and a model for more to come. It's jam up....beats anything you've ever seen. Old folks get sent there to play, not die.

Of course, we never know, but if he can continue to get better, life, though different can be fun.

In the meantime, my time is really strained, and of course, since I was basically broke before, well.... I can tell you this in the ICD format, because you are my friends. I still plan to get out the ICD, but my already eccentric schedule shall remain eccentric.

One thing that is quite important. If you do not receive the ICD for three months or so, give me a shout. It is not impossible that your name has been thwacked from my label base. I just dumped, well, actually, my 9 year old prodigy daughter just dumped all the names over to a database that works for a change, but just in case, if you don't hear from me in a reasonable length of time, let me know. Do not automatically assume that I've fled to Montana with the funds. Now, that's an idea!!

NEW FEATURE

Note on the bottom of your mailing label on your envelope a number. If you see one, you will see the last issue date on your subscription. Most of you old guys run out with 3-6. Until lately I've tried to keep everybody on the same track, but due to increased readership, different folks will run out at different times.

You can see when to re-up by studying that label. A subject that I've given a great deal of thought to since starting the ICD was "What exactly is its place in ICdom?"

For no particular reason, I think I'll elucidate. Imagine if you will, war in the Pacific, 1943. The fleet, which is made up of many ships is steaming around, doing battle here and yon. Our task force is made up of lesser ships, a battle wagon, and a little mail boat. I see the ICD as the little mail boat that could. You, my friends are the lesser ships.

Sometimes, I get jaded to the fact that I'm dealing with the creme of the crop. For each of you, there are 40 more who really couldn't care less about the cause, and no amount of prodding is going to change that statistic. Then, there is the XXX, which I liken to the battleship. A ponderous thing, she takes in a wide circle, and is slow of movement sometimes, but oh my, let her bring her guns to bear, and a mighty lady she is!

Then, there is the little mail boat, bringing news to all the other ships at sea. The ICD is that little boat. That's all it wants to be, all it ever will be. But isn't it nice to get mail from home?

Speaking of newsletters. Lately I have gotten two letters expressing the same sentiment. There is concern over the format of the ICD....not content...format. I'll be the first to admit that it might not be the easiest thing around to read. The reason for the look you see this month is that I try to jam pack as much info as possible into as little paper as possible. Course, this makes for eyestrain. We have several possibilities: 1. Keep it as is. 2. Go to standard size type. 3. Go to standard size type and 6 pages instead of 4 and charge 10 bucks a year.

Since I can vouch for the fact that there are po' folks out there, I hesitate on option 3, but it is your call. If I get enough feedback, I will make a format change. If not, it will stay the same.

It's your call. Let me know what you think, before the next issue. Additionally, and thanks to AJ in Wisconsin, I'll be using the updated version of my word processing program, which mainly offers more graphics, and tonite I will order an extra printer ribbon that will be used exclusively for the ICD...(darker print!) This stuff ain't cheap. Again, our thanks to angel #1, AJ.

Back in May of this year, Dr. Fugazotto, our American urinary researcher spoke before the XXX at their meeting in New Orleans...at the risk of his fragile health I am told. He had only a short address, much too short, but of great import to our needs. He said that our urinary culturing methods are fine for the standard types of infection that they are geared to detect, but fail, utterly, in the face of something outside the parameters, ergo, IC infection detection.

In the last edition of the ICD, I touched base on the research being conducted overseas, research into UTI (Urinary Tract Infection) that dated back to 1984, research that could have, by now, revolutionized the methods of detection and treatment of IC. To tell you the truth, I intended to get really pig out on this super glut of info Judy M and Ruth K from VA. sent. However, after reading an article sent to me by Rosalind Maskell of Portsmouth, England, I decided to go about it another way I'll mention shortly.

I received letter a from Rosalind Maskell, one of the British authors of the search for UTI dated July 3rd. It was a polite, but short letter, and seemed relatively unimpressed that we too were on the bacterial track for IC. Also there was no recognition of the fact that I relayed a message from the NIH that American funding could very well be made available upon request.

Researchers universally keep their cards close to their vests. Not to get the wrong idea, I am happy just to hear from a big name scientist, by golly. The ICD is after all, not JAMA.(Journal of Medical something or other.)

Alright. Rosalind Maskell sent two articles. One was from the JOURNAL OF INFECTION, (1989),19 and the other from the BRITISH JOURNAL OF UROLOGY,(1989),64.

Although one article is exclusively dedicated to IC and the Urethral Syndrome, the other, which is called "A new look at the diagnosis of infection of the urinary tract and its adjacent structures" is the better of the two.

Frankly, the work is so well done, that for me to try and paraphrase it, as I usually try to do, would be an injustice to you the reader. There is so much info packed into these pages that I just don't dare try. Again, thanks to Judy M and Ruth K, I am privy to the articles that led up to this treatise, and I can tell you that this one really sums things up.

To highlight, Rosalind Maskell speaks of the history of our current methods of urinalyses, speaks to its weaknesses as far as a predictor in oddball cases like our IC, delves into electron micropsy and its pictures of microorganisms embedded in the bladder.....Speaks to men with chronic prostatitis about the bacterial connection, even chides doctors a bit about not being more precise in their wants and needs from the lab.

Rosalind Maskell defines our kind of bugs as fastidious bacteria, and says they may be defined as organisms "which require cultural conditions other than overnight incubation in air on a primary isolation medium."

If you recall from that most popular of ICD's on Urinary Sampling Techniques, a while back, Rosalind Maskell speaks to standard cultures on an agar medium. Rosalind Maskell makes what would have been a year ago (In IC time), a sad observation, "—exhaustive searches for causes of inflammation other than infection have been unsuccessful."

Today, however, in the IC world, we are getting used to shocks much as if it were simply another communist country hanging their leader.

There is much more. As much as I hate to say to you that you should send more money, I must at this time do that very thing. Since this article is so good, and is written in doctor language, and would make a wonderful offering for your favorite medical person, I will make copies available for $5 bucks a throw.

You get 10 pages, front and back mailed to your door. This will cost at least $3.50 to 4 bucks, so if I do, say 10 copies, the ICD can pocket the diff. If you want a copy, let me know. It's the closest thing we have to an inspired document at this time as far as IC goes. To make it easier on me, please send me your request plus 5 bucks before the second week in September, at which time I will process all the requests at one time. If you are reading this magazette much later, don't worry, I'll make you a copy if you want it....however, things are moving so fast, just about the time we digest one bit of good news, another comes along to put the last in the shade!

In summation, it looks like Rosalind Maskell and Fugazotto agree that in many cases, IC is caused by a bacterial agent. Current American literature defines IC as an ill defined condition for which no cause has been found and no effective therapy developed. If we have to do it one doctor at a time, let's get the word out that there is indeed a possible definition of IC, and that definition is good ol' bacterial infection.

Let's check the mail............

Pearl P of Carlisle, Pa. writes," My urologist, who has been treating me for the past 3 years was not impressed with Dr. F.'s findings. In fact, he did a culture again and said the bacteria Dr. F. found was not found in the culture....

" OK....I don't know the particulars of Pearl's doc's methods, and I AM NOT a doctor, but see, you can't find the bacteria that Dr. Fugazotto is seeing and that Rosalind Maskell has been seeing with standard methods. It just doesn't work.

If you did see Gardnerella vaginalis as Rosalind Maskell calls it, or gaffkya as Dr. F. says, then their work would be all wrong. Rosalind Maskell cultures her stuff in a 7% carbon dioxide atmosphere and Dr. F. uses a broth culture medium. Neither of these methods are routinely, if ever, employed in a standard lab.

Pearl goes on to say that she has tried Dr. F.'s treatment and had to stop because her antibiotic did not agree with her tummy. We know what you mean, Pearl. Just about anyone with IC has problems with drugs. Frankly, that was why I was so surprised that I could tolerate Augmentin so well. Thanks for writing, Pearl, and your info is on the way. Pearl was to receive some information that I had from earlier medical forays, but will now be the first to get the above mentioned report from Rosalind Maskell.

Just received a letter from Doris T in Scottsdale, AZ. Yep, we're out west now....I'll tell you how in a couple of lines... Doris says that she has had IC since Oct of 1987. She has tried Dr. F.'s recommendations starting back in April. Everything improved greatly for awhile and then she had a relapse. On the road to it she developed a yeast infection, but beat it. She says that she's going to be in the good doctor's area and will visit him and Georgia.

Yes, Georgia is back, but only part-time, maybe. Much conflicting news about the gal. I got the idea from the exclamation marks on someone's letter that Ga. may have got mad at me for reporting that she had split in an earlier ICD. Oh well....as long as I don't have to go to jail for libel.....Can I help it if you are becoming legend by association? Super thanks for writing, and when you see some of your other out west IC friends, like in the next state, tell them about the ICD.

Yvonne R of York Pa. gets an ICD angel award this issue. She has written a couple or three very nice letters, and sent at least 3 more IC buddies my way. She is the founder of our move across the Mississippi! She's been out in Phoenix getting a little sun all summer but should be back in Pa. when this thing runs... Yvonne says that Phillip H..., one of the old guard IC researchers who resides in Philly said in Emergency Magazine 6-15-89, that in 1915, Hunner. (of Hunner.'s ulcers fame...an old name for IC) said that IC arose from chronic bacterial infection.

The problem with this is that just lately we have come to the conclusion, quite apart from current medical thinking, that you have to treat chronic bacterial infection with chronic medication. A two week dosage just doesn't get it. A doc will issue the standard course, and of course, no results, or very little. That's the theory anyway...again, I must remind you to remember that we are at the very start of a possible breakthrough. Do what your doctor says, and if you don't like what he says, get another. We are, after all amateurs.

Yvonne also mentions that she has been taking medication for 8 months and is doing well...One problem is, that we don't know when to stop. So much research to be done yet! Hang in there Yvonne.

Many writers have enquired about my health. Well, several months ago, I was in the hospital for a checkup. I had been on Augmentin for a month and a half and was developing some pretty IC pains after a stint of great health. I decided to go off the day of the tests, which turned out ok.

Frankly, I was about dead, eat up with IC symptoms, caused by the medication. While the doc was looking, I had him pump me up with DMSO laced with Kennalog/Heparin. Normally, I don't personally go in for such things, but I theorized that just maybe, since my system was saturated with antibiotics, particularly the urine, the DMSO might wash some of it into the tissue. Kinda like a penetrating bug spray! It must have worked. After I nearly had a lower torso fit tossing off the treatment or x-ray dye, or GREAT TASTING laxative, or whatever, for 3 days afterwards, bango, I felt great...could sit comfortably, the works.

Course, my ol' bladder is so far gone that I didn't have much of a capacity change, but the frequency seemed to improve, and I slept better. It's just my little pet theory, but, maybe DMSO might be best used to help transport the antibiotics through the tissues to the infection. Liken it to mixing weed spray with kerosene. It's just my theory. If you have a chance to ever test it, for gosh sakes let me know if you see an improvement.

Everything went well until my father had the stroke and I guess the stress caused me to slide. I'm taking Augmentin again, and so far so good. Stress definitely is a factor with IC, I think it's safe to say.

Judy M, our super sleuth from VA. writes. She sends her best to all and a daily IC chart form to help you with your home research. She and her husband devised it and I must say, it has one I came up with a while back beat all to heck. The form will be included with the Rosalind Maskell papers. Many, many thanks from a devoted ICD crew!!!

One note here regarding last issue's report of intravenous medication. I know some forms of it exist, because I've had it as far back as 1972. However, at present I don't have any info as to what is or is not available, particularly as pertains to our latest antibiotic weapons as specified by Dr. F. I haven't heard from anyone on actual experiments with IV antibiotics yet, but it remains a tantalizing prospect for the future...

Several issues ago I made a statement that I felt that there existed on-shelf technology that could in some way help with our IC problem. Judy M found that technology in the form of some dusty British musings dating back to 1984, if you recall from above. I have a confession to make. When I made that statement, I was actually thinking of stomach ulcers. It seems like our problems are similar. Well, guess what....from OMNI, August 1990 comes word that, "The most common cause of these stomach disturbances (ulcers) is a corkscrew shaped microorganism called Helicobacter pylori, which borrows into the wall of the stomach, making victims susceptible to virtually any irritant."

What does this mean to us? You extrapolate it.

Last issue, I reported on a letter from Marjorie P way up yonder in Canada. She raises an interesting point. What of long term antibiotic treatment? I profess that it scares me, but not quite as badly as IC. Further she said that she is trying Trinalin, which I reported helped me. Trinalin, if you recall is an antihistamine. Normally, I can't even take an aspirin, so I was quite vividly surprised that I could tolerate it so well, and that it actually moderates my IC.

Of course, even with the best of miracle drugs in you, you just have to watch what you eat! You are what you eat, and I guarantee you that if you are anywhere near an end-stager like me a taco can make you wish for morphine. So, back to long term antibiotics.....I just don't know. Read the fine print on the pamphlet you can get, or in the Physician's Desk Reference, and proceed. You are what you eat, and that includes antibiotics. We are in Indian Territory now. Anything is possible....streams strangled with beaver, or trouble around the bend. However this turns out, at the least, I think our children will be much more prepared for life with IC thanks to us pioneers.

(**Editor note<2014>:** See, even back then I knew we were pioneers!)

Dixie K, one of our oldest ICD'ers reports in....She says that she has been antibiotic free for 3 months now after the Dr. F. diet and is still doing well. Great going! She sends me a copy of a page from one of the British articles dug up by Judy M. I already have it...but it is instructive to know that the good news is spreading fast...however it is that you wound up with it....ooops, Judy M sent her the copy. Boy, that gal gets around. Thanks so much for writing, Dixie of Clinton, Ms. We can't hear from you often enough.

Ellen T from Bellvue Washington comes aboard. Can't get much further west than that. She fairly glows with compliments. My head already barely fits through the door now! Welcome, and if you get the chance, remember to spread the word about that ICD thing from the state where the residents go shoeless in the summer time.

Welcome aboard Celia L and Shirley C from Phoenix way, a-la Yvonne R. Celia sent me a copy of Dr. F.'s address to the XXX at the big meeting in May of 1990 for which I am very grateful. I sure didn't have it. This three page speech will be shrunken to fit on a single page and will accompany the Rosalind Maskell papers. Thanks so much Celia, and let your neighbors out in the wild west know about the ICD. (Boy, can I conjure up visions of her area!) I'm not very well traveled, you know.

AJ, God bless her, from Wisconsin writes. Holly, the state Coordinator, and super ICD'er has appointed her the assistant chief, and she's all fired up. AJ beat us all to the punch on something. Since it looks like IC may be of a bacterial nature, this opens up a whole new can of worms...to be precise, the Center for Disease Control (CDC) in Atlanta. Alice Jane has been corresponding with them.

I invite any and everybody to help AJ open them up on our behalf. Contact AJ at<address> , Wisconsin,. Really, this could mean a whole lot.....Would you believe that I was planning on visiting AJ on the second week of August. Well, due to our recent health problem, we had to very reluctantly scrap the trip. For me, going from Alabama to Wisconsin is like most of you going to Australia. Maybe next year.

(**Editor note<2014>:** One of my regrets to this day is that I never got to meet AJ, even though we almost made a trip to see her. A wonderful, wonderful woman!)

Isn't it funny how something like IC can make us almost family? There is more mail, and good mail, but my 'pooter says I'm all out or room. We have one more issue to get out in series by October, so we'll hopefully see you a little later. From Norman, Vicky, and of late, keypunchists C, and E, God bless you all, and keep digging. We are making progress...... Norm

The IC Disclaimer Issue 13

THE IC DISCLAIMER THE BIMONTHLY NEWSLETTER FOR INTERSTITIAL CYSTITIS
YOUR EDITOR: NORMAN MORRISON
THIS MONTH: "MAIL CALL AND MORE"

Greetings to all our new readers this issue. I think you will quickly find that you now belong to an extended family of IC'ers. Its pretty large, so there's always someone out there willing to help with information or just a friendly ear. The ICD is sort of a big ol' information clearinghouse.

Sometimes we have more information than we can deal with, at others, not enough. Right now this issue will be dedicated to catching up the mail.

First, a little business...and it's your fault. Last issue, I asked for feedback on a format change for the ICD. Well, starting next issue, you shall have your way. The ICD will go to 3 printed pages (six sides).

The original idea for the teeny type was to take a shortcut to pack as much text as possible into two pages. This hasn't worked out too well for some readers who don't possess a scanning electron microscope, so we'll be going back to standard sized text. The downside is that the price rises to 10 bucks a year to accommodate the extra page. This will cause untold amounts of confusion, so bear with us.

Until the recent influx of new readers the policy was to send back issues enough to make it to where everyone's subscription would come due in October. If you see a 3-6 on your mailing label, you should renew now for the next series. The ICD year starts in October. If you see, for example, a 4-5 on your label, then you know that your subscription expires with 4-5. You should send a check for (5 x 50 cents) or two dollars and fifty cents to cover our extra expense.

A handful of readers have a (cont) on their label. They receive the ICD free for various reasons.

(Editor note<2014>: Please bear with me here on the housekeeping. I suppose I was having all the fun using a brand new shiny database label printer. One of the first in existence for a home computer, actually. Earlier I made mention about my "keypunchist." That would be my daughter, who programmed the database for her old man. She could have been no older than 9 years old at the time. The E was my young son. I have no idea what part he played. I felt that it would be good training for them using computers to urge them to get involved)

See, I told you it would be confusing, and I've already taken up half this issue explaining it. Now you know what it means to change fish in mid-stream. So, in short, readers who are up with this issue need to renew at 10 bucks, and newer readers who expire sometime next year need to send in an extra check for the number of issues they have left at the rate of 50 cents apiece. Is this ridiculous or what? Bear with us for the next couple of months and we'll get square, and you'll get a better product. As always, if you have any questions, or problems, LET ME KNOW! We'll work it out. Also, if the new, higher rate is going to work a hardship on you, and you still want the ICD, let me know. We'll figger out something. In the meantime, be patient, and just remember that while confusion reigns, mistakes are bound to happen. We will work out of this, though. Nuff said.

There are two ways to slide easily through life; to believe everything or to doubt everything. Both ways save us from thinking.—-Alfred K.

Even if you're on the right track you'll get run over if you just sit there. -—Will Rogers

The IC DISCLAIMER is non-profit, but not tax deductible. One year costs $10.00. It is published 6 times a year. Please make your check payable to: Norm, the editor of this magazette. ..... Back issues as available are at regular prices.(3-3 forward..) Write. THANKS! All correspondence is considered public unless you specify otherwise. Your address may be made available to others with similar interests unless you say otherwise.*Your subscription expires with the number at the bottom of your mailing label.*KEEP WRITING!

After scanning the above text Vicky reminds me that I am not concise. So what's new?

Lately, we've been pretty single mindedly sticking to the Dr. Fugazotto-Rosalind Maskell theory of bacterial infection. Let's see what other theories-confirmations-whatever the mail brings.

Peggy T, Dover Pa....writes...(and just let me say right here, that everybody starts off by complimenting the ICD...which makes me extremely happy) that she's using something called Terazol to help prevent yeast infections while on Dr. Fugazotto's regimen.

I reckon everyone knows about Dr. F. by now. She says that her bladder is named Bart, and can be a bad puppy at times. She is also using an instilled substance called Sodium Cromalyn, or is it Sodium Cromoglycate, as the article (British Journal of Urology, (1986 58,95-96) by Edwards, Bucknall and Makin call it.

At this time, these guys said that they thought that IC was caused by a trauma (injury) to the bladder which released an "alteration to an antigen which reacts with immune-competent cells which may produce antibody. This in turn could cause more bladder damage and fibrosis. Injury, inflammation and fibrosis are parts of a self-perpetuating process."

The article goes on to say that out of 9 subjects studied, two had a complete resolution of IC. Two years later, one relapsed and one is still home free. A total of six out of the nine were helped. They admitted that they were a little disappointed.

Ah, readers, now this is more like the old ICD, before Dr. Fugazotto came along wrecking apple carts. The article goes on to describe their blend of secret herbs and spices. Peggy sent her own mixture which contains heparin, Nasalcrom, and Sensorcaine, which is instilled into the bladder and held for one hour.

If you want more info, I'm sure Peggy wouldn't mind corresponding with you. Your docs could get together. That's what info sharing is all about. As of July, Peggy was doing fine on her instillations and Dr. F. treatment. Not well, mind you, but much better. Oh yes...she said that a Chlorpactin infusion caused her much misery. Thanks for writing, Peggy. Let us here how everything is going.

Holly L, soul mate extraordinary, Menomonie, WI, writes that if she waited for the right or convenient time to write, I'd still be waiting. She had her bladder out several months ago, and as such, is an on-going test case for the rest of us on this procedure. Personally, I am aghast about it, but she puts up with me.

She attended the meeting in New Orleans a while back and she says she missed seeing two important figures in ICDOM, Ruth K from the Washington DC area and Melanie B, the SE coordinator.

More recently, I just spoke with AJ from Wisconsin, Holly's assistant coordinator, and ICD supporterwithoutequal.

Actually, AJ sends me in a few bucks extra, allowing me to do housekeeping chores like buying printer ribbons, word processor updates, and stamps, etc. (And tacking on extra pages!) Also, I lean on her quite a bit. Holly does too, because AJ said that she spent the night with her recently. They are great friends. They are, and we are, and you and I are great friends.

Holly is upbeat as usual, but AJ tells me that her Vulvitis has been kicking in. You might wish to send her a note of support, and any ideas that you may have on the subject. Thanks for writing Holly, and AJ.

Cindy-L A, Takoma Park, Maryland comes aboard with a letter, money, AND, a newsletter. She's the State Coordinator in that part of the world. You know...I can't really understand why someone would pick a silly name for their newsletter ....Just kidding, heh heh.

Silly names precede good information....From page one of THE BLADDERETTE #3........There are four stratum or coats that make up the wall of the bladder:

1. The mucosa is the innermost "coat". It is a mucous membrane containing transitional epithelium tissue which is able to stretch. The rugae are folds in the mucosa. Transitional epithelium tissue is special in that it is made up of large, round cells at its edge. This allows the tissue to be stretched or distended without the outer cells breaking apart from one another.

2. The submucosa is a layer of connective tissue that connects the mucosa and the muscular coats.

3. The detrusor muscle consists of three layers of smooth muscle [inner longitudinal, middle circular and outer longitudinal muscles.] [In the area around the opening around the urethra, the circular fibers form an internal sphincter muscle. Below the internal sphincter is the external sphincter, which is composed of skeletal muscle.]

4. The serous coat is formed by the peritoneum—the largest serous membrane of the body that lines the abdominal cavity and covers the organs.

Cindy says that the above has to do with the cystology of the bladder—-the study of tissues. She says that the next time your doc pulls histology on you, you can kind of non-chalantly, whilst checking your nails for lint or something, say, "Yeah, histology. I know what that is."

The Bladderette is an extremely well done newsletter, and I certainly hope that its readers in the Maryland area thank Cindy profusely because quality takes time. I hope she keeps me on her list. Hint hint. A careful reading of Cindy's report on bladder tissue will help you understand how Dr. Fugazotto's bugs can infiltrate your meaty parts, damage it and cause you much discomfort. Also, you'll see more clearly why it is so difficult to treat a deep seated infection. Many thanks to Cindy for an on-going job well done!

(Editor note<2014>: I could resist. I searched for The Bladderette on Google and found one reference. It got a mention in one of Dave Barry's columns of the day! Wow! If you don't know who Dave Barry is or was, then ask your mama or granny.)

A silly disclaimer here at this point from me. Many have requested back issues of the ICD and or information. On the latter. I am behind. That's the size of it. Some have been serviced, others not. If you haven't been answered, holler at me again. Frankly, I'm lost. Same with the back issues. If you have requested back issues and have not gotten them, let me know. You shall be rewarded for your patience. I haven't forgotten you. I can claim brain damage, probably from IC or something. It's the great blanket equalizer. So, if you need something, let me know again.

Donna S of Mo has written twice. Let's look at the more recent correspondence. Ah, a question on yeast. You might get in touch with Peggy on that score, or this dude below. At this point I will bravely try to insert some text from the ICD 2-2. Now, if this darn thing will just do it...(editor grunting presses several keys on the keyboard....) Time passes..... Ah Ha! It worked...From the ICD2-2........

* * *THE CASE OF LYNETTE SIGG * * * Several months ago, on my way to discovery, I ran across an article in an inspirational magazine by this young lady. Although the piece was primarily concerned with her journey of overcoming pain, it read like a typical case of IC. It took some doing, but I finally contacted her by mail, in Australia! I still can't say for sure that she had IC, but her description read like a textbook case. She claimed that she had overcame it. One of her weapons was the herb Slippery Elm which you can obtain at any health food store. Her recommendation was two tablets three times a day with meals. I tried it myself, and for a couple of weeks I felt tremendously better. Although it didn't affect the frequency it did nearly stop the pain. She stressed, however, that Slippery Elm only covers over the problems, and that only by going on an elimination diet can the cure begin. She gave me the titles of a couple of books, both by the same man, and would you believe that this author makes his home in Tennessee? Following out my lead I contacted the fellow; Dr.Crook, and he told me a bit about his work. It seems that he is currently working on the assumption that the yeast known as Candida Albicans(Did I say that right?) which can infest the human gut produces toxins that can cause a heck of a lot of discomfort down there. If you have had your lower intestines nearly catch on fire, or been suffering from pelvic pain in that region, you know what I'm talking about. Although he didn't seem to know much about IC, obviously the problems of Candida and food allergies can aggravate our IC. You see, what you eat can hit you immediately or 3 days later as it is processed and moved through the system. Further complicating the situation, there's not always a direct (Let me STRESS, in my opinion) correlation between what you eat and the symptoms. According to Crook, sugary foods aid the yeast infection which in turn introduces toxins into the system. These toxins can make you have watery eyes, they can elevate your blood pressure, they can give you diarrhea, or none of the above. On the other hand, you can be directly allergic to a food, and as it moves through the tubes give you a whole range of problems, or maybe this time nothing.

it's the darndest mess you've ever seen, but for many of us IC folks, it's our mess. Lynette Sigg, with the aid of a good allergy man said she overcame her problems. It might be a good area for us to look into problems, or maybe this time nothing. it's the darndest mess you've ever seen, but for many of us IC folks, it's our mess.

The information is still relevant...but my my, how far we have come. If you are interested in pursuing the yeast connection, contact Dr. Crook at PROFESSIONAL BOOKS, <Address>, or look for his books in the library...(doubtful), one in particular called TRACKING DOWN FOOD ALLERGY.

I talked to him, way back, and he was aware of IC, but that's about all. Yeast could, and may be a major factor in our problem, at least from the standpoint of our GI tract...at least that's where my thinking has evolved to date. Anyway, Donna, here it is.

Donna says hurrah to gaffkya being sexually transmitted. She says that her husband tested recently. His urine was negative but his semen was positive. Take note, gentlemen with IC AND prostate problems. She also says Georgia told her about the ICD. Many thanks to the elusive Georgia. Somebody please make sure that Georgia gets copy of he ICD... Everybody has a different idea on Georgia's disposition. Is she working, not working, or going to work for Dr. F. I, Norman Morrison, just remain confused. Hope springs eternal though...in a moment....

A clarification. Donna asks about something in the last issue of ICD. OK...The British have been working to a purpose on bacteria and IC since 1984. They culture the little buggers under a carbon dioxide atmosphere. They call their bugs, Gardenerella vaginalis (quoting from Donna's spelling.)

Dr. Fugazotto, on the other hand who was working on the same problem since around 1964 and cultures his critters with a broth medium calls his pets, Gaffkya. There is no possible way to tell, till they get together, if they get together, but they may indeed be looking at the same bacteria.

To me, one is round, one is rod shaped and one is squiggly. I rest my case on my expertise.(* Ah dear reader....see the difference a day can make....we'll come back to this issue on the lastpage....Ed.)

Donna mentions antihistamines. She thinks that's how her problem started. One of my many theories about myself includes the usage of one of those 12 hour nose openers. At the least, I know now that it will open more than your nose, if you have IC. Was it a contributing factor...I don't know, but it is a personal suspect. Mucous is mucous, whether it be in the nose, or elsewhere.

Oddly enough, I have, as mentioned in an earlier edition, I had some success with an antihistamine called Trinalin. It opens my nose, though it makes me drowsy as all get out, and ameliorates the effects of certain biological irritants like mold and grass spores, and some food problems, should I get into something that I shouldn't have.

I only take it when absolutely necessary. Again, this is strange, since I can't even stand an aspirin. Haven't heard from anyone else who's tried it yet. Again, one man's pepper upper is another's botulism extract. Be very cautious when sampling any new medication. Use common sense, and your doc's close guidance. Thanks again, Donna! We'll be looking to hear more from you.

Linda B from Seattle comes aboard. She says to drink lots of water. Welcome aboard, and you are on the 10 buck list already. Did you get a back issue on Dr.F. from me? Hmm. See what I mean? What with all this talk of Dr. Fugazotto, you might be wondering what the old boy looks like. I had the pleasure to meet with him several months ago, so I know. Georgia, on the other hand remained a pleasant mystery, a young woman cloaked in legends coat almost as much as the good doctor.....

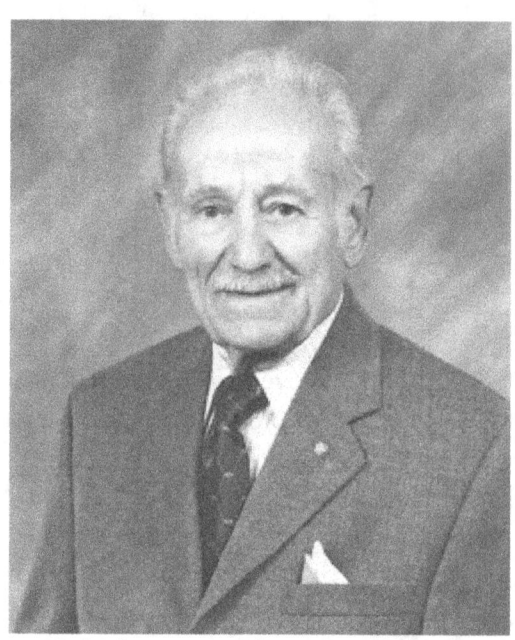
Dr. Fugazzotto in his later years. Photo supplied by David Fugazzotto

Well, thanks to Doris T, our questions have now been answered. Elsewhere in this document, behold the good doctor and his assistant. Sounds kinda like an opener for an old radio play. It's easy enough to thwack down a picture and copy it, of course it comes out a little funky. It's a bit harder to get it to come out looking right, and a lot more expensive. Thanks go to AJ and her helping ways to allow us all to see our friends in Rapid City.

Doris and her husband arrived in South Dakota on July 29th and snapped this picture for us after taking a 5000 mile round trip tour around the country. They live in Scottsdale, Az. She writes that she was very impressed with both Dr. F. and Georgia and visited with them for two hours. She stated what I think is all our wishes, that Dr. Fugazotto someday gets proper recognition for his pioneering research into the cause and cure for IC.

Doris asks about antibiotics causing irritation to the bladder. It has been my experience, and others as well, that many foods and other substances irritate the bladder. Antibiotics are no exception. I can, for example, tolerate Augmentin for no longer than a month and a half, then the side effect of irritation begins to overshadow the curative quality. I can't even take an aspirin without risk of inflaming the bladder. As I postulated in an earlier ICD, I believe that as your IC becomes more advanced, so does your tendency toward food and substance sensitivity.

Coffee, tea, and chocolate seem to be the first things to go, followed by many other foods. Heck, I nearly died from a case of acute squash poisoning early in the summer. I love the little yellow buggers fried up golden brown, but that love is not returned. Just as with tomatoes, at least in my case, it looks like the seeds are the culprit.

(Editor note<2014>: Tomatoes are still a problem. However my most recent major discovery was that mustard really ramps up my IC. Yes, yellow mustard!)

But, back to antibiotics....Personally, there are many that I can't take now. Luckily, and surprisingly, Augmentin is still fairly tolerable to me. Since this area is so new, I'm afraid conjecture is all we have. This, I THINK, points to an information void. As good as Dr. F.'s treatment is, I think that he would be the first to agree that basically we are just getting started.

He has only a few antibiotics to work with and only in pill form. Speculation is that IV antibiotic treatment would be much better. Maybe there will come even a better way. Right now we don't have IV antibiotics to mention. (Well maybe one or two, but I don't know enough on the subject to even mention it yet.)

I don't even think that we have the RIGHT antibiotics. The problem is that a lot of research has to go into the development and testing of these drugs and right now IC is just under belly button lint on the list. The idea is to find a drug specific for a given infection.

Like Dr. F. says, traditional shot in the dark medications and short duration runs can actually aggravate the problem. Dr. F. has come up with the best list of specifics he can find today. The goal is to come up with even better ones, and/or better ways of delivering it.

Doris says that she had a lovely conversation with Donna S down in MO after finding out about her in an earlier ICD. That's the ICD at its best. Doris says finally that she has flare-ups occasionally. I know this is probably going to go over like a (You fill in the blank), but are you watching that diet?

There are all sorts of things like grass pollen, mold spores, you name it, lurking out there anyway, but new food sensitivities happen from time to time. Doris is no piker, so I'm sure she knows all about this sort of thing....but I had to ask, just the same. There may be a newer IC victim out there somewhere not so aware of the food connection. We are what we eat. Super thanks for the pic of our favorite scientists, Doris!

From Anne E, ,York Harbor, Maine ...Boy, some people have all the luck!

"Where you live at Norm?"

"Alabama"...

"Oh, too bad..."

Boy, Maine, now there's a state for you. Everything up there is some kind of harbor, and they have nor'easters and such. AND its not 100 degrees 3 months out of the year! Be that as it may, Anne has a serious request. She says that she's looking for folks who have or know about a condition called FIBROMYALGIA/FIBROCYTIS which is also similar to Polymyalgia Rheumatica. (Holly?)

She says that it is characterized by tender points on the body, usually elbows, back, chest, stiffness, pain in the arms, legs, back, shoulders, fatigue, sleeplessness, along with good old irritable bowel syndrome. She says that the AMA in their journal devoted the entire Feb 1986 issue to it. She says her doc thinks it may be connected to the immune system, and may even be related to IC.

This is a new one on me. If you identify with this problem please drop Anne a line. Also, let me know. Every connection we make furthers the cause, because there ain't no them, it's only us doing the work right now, dear readers. Let us know how it goes Anne...and thanks!

From Carmela W, Nashua, New Hampshire.... Carmela says she was diagnosed in the early seventies. She said that two years ago she was about ready to throw in the towel and have out with the bladder. Her doc talked her into trying the Hemlstein procedure. (I ought to know what that is, but at the moment it escapes me.) and alcohol cytolysis, which has to do with the dissolution of certain nerves in the bladder.

She says she is not cured, but was much helped. Different strokes, as they say. I know this technology has been around for some time. If you have tried this, or are interested, Carmela says to write or call if you'd like to hear her story. Thanks much Carmela, and thanks for sharing your approach with us. It's the foundation of the ICD.

I received around the middle of August a letter from one of the ICD's oldest customers, and a right smart check to boot. Jan J from Mississippi way writes that her daughter just got married in June (naturally) and she actually even likes her son-in-law. Hmm...I should wish a dose of IC on my mother-in-law if this kind of behavior is common with the afflicted. She's not nearly so nice as Jan.

She also said that her home is on a "historic homes" tour. Mine is too. Our house is considered an antique in the "early depression" tradition. Ha.

Perhaps Jan has discovered the best method of infiltrating the doctorgensia...she's sending her son to medical school.... Just about when you thought we were at least winning the PR war with physicians Jan tells a tale of a young woman down in her area who recently went to a doctor who assured her that she was indeed crazy and needed a psychiatrist. Worse, he convinced her family of that fact.

Jan asks me to warn you about this guy, but my limited better sense says whoa up. Want to hear a good old fashioned IC horror story? Give Jan a shout at <address> MS.

I've had some corny moments with docs who couldn't figure out my mystery malady, but nothing out and out classically bad. Particularly, if you are in the Mississippi area, you might do well to get a line on this. Jan hadn't written in a while and was worried that we might have forgotten about her. No way Jan!! Good to hear from you.

One small note from me...Last issue I reported that I father had a stroke. Well, we have him in a nursing home now, a super nice one. Things have stabilized somewhat, though we are rife with paperwork and bills. Life goes on, though a bit more stressfully. We'll make it. You don't know how much your words of encouragement mean to us...Thanks.

Well, we come to the end of another ICD. For me its time to spell check, revise and add graphics, plus figure out where to put that pretty picture of Dr. F. and Georgia. Next issue comes in the new format and the new price. I kinda got used to getting around in this format, so it will be a challenge the next time around. If you feel shorted, cheated, forgotten, miffed, whatever, drop me a note. Changing over is going to be fun! We aims to please. Remember to watch what you eat, and don't forget that God is another way of saying good. Whatever the state of your faith, right now is the time to be as far as IC research goes.

If we stick to our guns maybe our kids won't be under the IC gun. Take care, and we'll see you next issue. IS IT GARDNERELLA OR GAFKYA?

Hello again on page five. I have a little more info that just came in plus some stuff I just thought of. Call it an end of the year blow out.

You can expect the Rosalind Maskell papers about two weeks after you receive this issue of the ICD..(Sept 1990.) If you are just coming aboard, the Rosalind Maskell papers is a copy of some of this British researcher's latest work on their version of bacterial infection and IC, plus a couple of other things.

If you want it, please send 5 bucks post haste to cover duplication and mailing. Just about the time you thought it was safe to write -finis- , well, here comes something else.

THERE IS ANOTHER. Meaning that there is another fired up chapter about to come into the IC fold. I want to welcome my super new friends from the San Antonio gang. I hope you find something new or interesting in the ICD. Special thanks goes to Jan K, San Antonio, TX for sending me massive amounts of annotated info on just about everything going on in their neck of the woods.

We'll be looking into that in the next issue. If you've noticed in this issue, I've included quite a few addresses. There is a reason. Reason one is that most of us want to hear from others, but reason two is that especially since Judy M came up with the Rosalind Maskell info, Ruth and the VA gang met with Dr. Fugazotto, the news has for the most part overwhelmed the ICD. There seems to be an amazing amount of things going down out there. Things are happening faster than the ICD can report. All I've done lately is grab onto what I could and hang on for the ride. When I say welcome aboard, you'd better be running if you want to get on.

Things are stirring out in ICLand! The giant is about to sit up. Things are no where near as simple for the ICD as they were a year ago. Who do I have to thank (or blame) for this...valiant government researchers? National press? Huge associations? Nope...just little groups out there plugging away, fighting, scratching and clawing in their own manners to further IC research.

Well, anyway, I wanted you to know that things are getting pretty frantic just about now. A tip from the ICD crystal ball. After Ruth and the gang in Virginia who have been in business these several months working on Dr. F. research, look west to Phoenix. (Super thanks to Yvonne R for colonizing this great group for the ICD!!!) I talked with Celia L and then Trish S the Arizona State XXX Coordinator called me.

Though I never figured out quite how, they seem to be well up on just about everything going on in the IC research field. They are planning to have Dr. Fugazotto as a speaker on October 7th and according to these young ladies they are looking for two blow-out sessions. The seating is limited to 45 per session and guess what? Doctors and such will be taking up a lot of that space!

Celia tells me that response has been great. If you just might happen to be jetting around the area about then you can RSVP a seat by contacting Trish at (X) in Phoenix. See what I mean? It's just getting bigger and better all the time.....and then there is the San Antone group. I've just been contacted, so I don't have any details, but it looks good...real good. I wonder what other surprises are in store for us?

Okay....I want to extricate my feets from my mouth which were liberally inserted last issue. I said that I felt like Dr. Fugazotto figured standard culturing techniques as seen in labs around the country was fine for standard kinds of infections. Celia L and Donna S said they didn't agree with that interpretation. Donna backed it up with some new info. Alright, maybe it was me that figured that standard lab techniques are good for standard infections.

Dr. Fugazotto sure as heck doesn't. In retrospect, from my lofty perch of commenter, I suppose I was speaking about common, easily treatable buggers, the kind most folks get and get rid of. What I didn't stop to consider is that even though Ms. Doe gets rid of a light case of cystitis, Gaffkya could still be lurking down there, unrevealed by standard approaches.

Dr. Fugazotto describes the current UTI approach thusly, "tests focused on finding urinary contaminants rather than pure culture etiologic agents-."

I think Dr. Fugazotto feels like one Gaffkya bug is as good as a herd. Standard procedures only recognize herds. The ICD, issue 3-3 covered standard techniques pretty thoroughly. I was extremely impressed with the technology in issue 3-3. Now, I don't know. I do have a problem with one thing though...If you toss out the standard culturing method...then what? Are there enough trained microbiologists to go around? One guy can oversee hundreds of samples a day using the regular approach. To implement the kind of change in UTI diagnosis looks to me like you are talking about yet another revolution.

Can IC'ers support two revolutions? We already have one going. Boy, I kinda wish for the days when all I had to worry about was whether or not white chocolate was safe to eat. Remember sun tea? That was a good one. I think that for the time being, perhaps we could compromise by educating the physicians. For example, if a doctor does a culture on a cystitis patient and it comes back negative, or the patient does not get better, then move on to more intensive techniques, namely Dr. F.'s method.

Right now, when someone obviously has a UTI problem and the sample shows no growth what's the doc to do. You know what. Every ICD reader has a story or two....What do you think?

Finally, for crying out loud....Donna S wrote a while back with a question, and then went and got it answered, or maybe looked after would be a better term. The answer to the question just makes more questions. Donna made a connection. I said last issue that perhaps Maskell's bacteria and Dr. F.'s bacteria were the same thing. So much for conjecture....

Quoting from Dr. Fugazotto's answer to Donna,"Gardernerella vaginalisas is a Gram variable bacillus found in vaginal discharge. Gaffkya is a Gram-positive coccus appearing in the lab in groups of (Gaffkya tetragena). These two organisms are not the same. I have not, to my knowledge, encountered Gardnerella in UTI's."

Donna wants to know if we are seeing two different organisms. Well, are we? I sure don't have the answer. If you have ordered the latest Rosalind Maskell tracts, I think you will find that she and Fugazotto's work compliments each other very nicely, all except the problem that she calls it one thing and Dr. Fugazotto calls it something else. Somebody has to lose on this one. Happily, I believe the IC'ers of both countries will come out winners.

One last note. Donna and I agree that the Center for Disease Control in Atlanta is ripe for picking. Be sure to put them on your mailing list. With their resources, if we can get them interested....well, you can see the potential.....

Many thanks to super ICD supporter, Donna S. She and many of my readers say many nice things about the ICD. Like I told her, the feeling is reciprocated. For all of you amateur scientists out there, just know that YOU have a fan....ME and the ICD! Well, I just got off the phone with a young fellow from Virginia who is wondering if he has IC. I told him what I knew and sent him to Dr. Fugazotto. Friends, it never ends. It never ends unless we end it. The future is in our hands. Work hard.

The IC Disclaimer Issue 14

THE IC DISCLAIMER THE BIMONTHLY MAGAZETTE FOR INTERSTITIAL CYSTITIS

YOUR EDITOR:Norm

THIS MONTH: A New Year Of Hope

(Editor note<2002>: The ICD ran through Issue 5-1 but we stop here.)

I want to extend a hearty welcome to the new readers of the ICD, and a long over due hello to all my old buddies. To tell the truth, I've been pretty busy these last couple of months. I'll leave it at that, cause, should I dig into my bag of excuses, we could be here for quite some time.

Anyways, this issue marks the start of the '91 ICD season. Lately, I've taken to getting business out of the way first. First, my apologies to about 3 users who did not get the last issue, Combo 3-6/4-1.

The fact is that I knew someone was lacking because the letters came back with the labels missing. I know what happened, so this shouldn't happen again. I don't even have a copy for myself. There are no whole back issues of any kind available. You will get the text of the issue without the little graphic doo-dads. I hope this will get you by.

On this subject, I will make available to anyone who wants it, all back issues. All it takes to get them is a computer with a modem. You can have any and all ICD's for the phone call. If interested, let me know. Somebody in your support group should be able to take me up on the offer.

We go to the new format with this issue...larger print and more pages. Boy, I've been dreading this first one, because it takes some more fiddling to know when to quit writing. The price has gone up to 10 bucks, as you know. For those of you who came in at the old price, don't worry about it. Our funds are looking pretty good right now, thanks to a little extra help from some of the ICD supporters.

We'll make it. In the little time the ICD has been off the air, much information has come in. Most of it is nothing new and astounding, but interesting. Of course, if you are new to the ICD, some of this may well be astounding. For example, for some time, the ICD has come down on the side of Dr. Fugazotto.

We think he has discovered the cause and cure of IC. Whoa now, back up a little. There is an insidious root cause for our problem that still exists, we think, for there is some reason we go on to get it and others don't. But for the new readers, it goes something like this: Everyone has bacteria in the bladder. Most are good little buggers, or at least not offensive. Some can cause cystitis. One type in particular called Gaffkya has been implicated as being the bug that starts eating away at the inner lining of our bladders, allowing urine to contact the meaty parts, causing scarring, pain, etc. Chances are that a lot of people are walking around with Gaffkya and never have a problem. We, the lucky, the few, however, welcomed them to our bladder bosoms with open ureters, where they proceed to chomp at us even as we read this text.

Conventional urine culturing techniques fail to reveal the vicious little buggers, so we don't get the proper medicine to combat the plague. Dr. Fugazotto, ICdom's patron saint, worked out a way to grow the vermin, and thus to identify them as our problem. Further, he worked out the best antibiotic course and length of treatment.

Fugazotto, basically, was discovered just a couple of years ago, so it will take some time for his pioneering research to filter down to local doctors. There is some work being done here and there around the country on his findings, but relatively speaking, very little. All work that is being done was spurred by our amateur researchers, many who subscribe to the ICD.

As stated many times before, there ain't no them out there, only us. I had a chance, once again to meet with the good doctor in January of this year. As per usual, he was flat on his back. He was having some work done on his leg to improve the blood flow. We met for about 20 minutes at UAB in Birmingham.

I must say that even groggy, he's the nicest fellow you'd ever want to meet. He was sporting a plethora of wires connected all over his body. Heck, he even had some kind of light on one of his finger nails. Downright strange! I have heard, since, from the S's that he has already returned to the lab...(Feb 91) and is much improved.

He sent the ICD some of his latest prose, namely to the Southern Medical Journal, who is quite interested in his work. Also, and I must chuckle loudly, thus breaking my stoic profile, he sent me a copy of a letter he sent to the XXX regarding his trip to New Orleans, among other things.

To put it mildly, he blasted them for their stance on his research. Many of the rank and file out there profess consummate confusion at the inability of the XXX to come to terms with his research, (As well as that of the British who have been working along similar lines since 1984) and concrete support of time worn treatments and studies, whose value, quite frankly, in light of our new information is about as useful as dinosaur scat.

The last thing the ICD wants to do is to divide the opinion of its readers, because a group divided can be conquered, but I've about had it folks. It's about time that the battlewagon of our fleet turns its guns on the real enemy, and that enemy is the pathogenic cause of IC. Enough time has been wasted in observing what the bacteria do. Let's start getting rid of them so we won't have any occasion to visit their damage.

THE LARGER PROBLEM: I don't want to spend too much time on this, but, dear readers, in the days since we last chatted, something finally soaked into my brain. Dr. Fugazotto's larger mission is to let the world know that there is a problem in Urinary-Land. Whenever you go to the hospital, the first thing they do is have you tinkle into a bottle. Many wondrous things can be divined from your specimen. On the chemical side, for instance, they can quickly tell if you have diabetes. As to bacteria, well, that's a different story.

The problem is not that the tests are inaccurate, but that they are incomplete. Modern technology looks for a relatively large grow-out of bacteria before it pronounces you infected. Dr. Fugazotto has found that standard methods won't grow out Gaffkya, therefore, you are pronounced bacteria free.

Chances are that there may be other types of organisms that don't respond to current techniques. He says that instead of relying on a large presence of bacteria, all it takes to prove that you have an infection is just two or three of the little fellers. For this work, you have to rely on the microscope, plus a few special growing techniques. Chances are that if this protocol had been used, you may not have gone on to the situation you are in now, because you may have received the right and proper treatment in the beginning of your IC.

Chances are that there are other problems out there, besides IC that aren't being found because of the methods employed in labs around this country. Fugazotto is out to change the very face of this bedrock lab work. As you can see, he's after larger fish than just IC, but in the process, has given us a better chance to lick our problem than has come along in the last 90 years.

Dr. Fugazotto with a little help from his friends made two tapes a few months ago. I'm sure that they will be eye-openers not only for you but your doctor as well. To tell you the truth, he gives enough examples of proof of his work to make you want to gag. It goes on and on.... These tapes are NOT recommended for a cozy evening in front of the microwave. However, they are required viewing for anyone who seriously wants to get something done.

If money is short I would recommend tape #2 over tape #1, however, both should be gotten if possible. My copy is being reviewed by a local hospital lab worker even as you read this....This will be the first stop in my projected tour.

#1 Detection Of Urinary Tract Infection

#2 Classical Technology For Identifying Causes Of Urinary Tract Infections.

Much, much work was put into this project by the producers, much volunteer work. It was conceived and done for the best of all reasons, to help strangers. Perhaps, one of these days, I'll be able to tell you their story.

The IC DISCLAIMER is non-profit, but not tax deductible. One year costs $10.00. It is published 6 times a year. Please make your check payable to: Norman , the editor of this magazette...... Back issues as available are at regular prices. Write first. THANKS!

All correspondence is considered public unless you specify otherwise. Your address will be made available to others with similar interests unless you say otherwise.*Your subscription expires with the number at the bottom of your mailing label.*KEEP WRITING! MAIL!

Everyone's mail contains money writs! They have just been cashed, finally. Some go back to the last flood! If you recall, much to the dismay of my wife, I hold money from issue to issue.

Whenever I wait 3 months, whew! I mean well, anyway.

*From Pearl C. , PA. Pearl says she hopes my father is doing well. He had a stroke in July, and we had to put him in a nursing home. I have worked for him in our electrical business for the last 8 years, so many problems had to be overcome. Everything, while not as we would like them, are better now. Thanks, all for your support!

Pearl says that she relies on Amitryptiline for relief, and it is helping. You know that I tried the stuff and couldn't hack it. Sent me off into nungy land. I'm one of those guys they wrote the *Exceptions* part about on the little sheet that comes with the bottle. For some, it has helped.

You might recall that I have found the antihistamine Trinalin quite helpful at times. Like amitryptiline, it doesn't help everyone. God bless you too, Pearl! Thanks for the mail.

Personally, on Fugazotto's regime, seems like I get about 6 months of excellent relief, (though I still have to go about as often) then lapse back. I'm trying to save up a little poke so I can afford to go back on his recommended antibiotic for a month or so. Done it twice so far.

*Welcome to Rosalyn J and Dr. James R Austin, TX.

* Carol H B, Newark, wrote a super letter. Seems like she's really been through the ringer. She asks about allergies and IC, which is one of my favorite topics. The ICD used to say that IC may be caused by allergies, way back in the before-time. Indeed, allergies may be the root cause of our problem, irritating our bladders, allowing the Gaffkya to get a start, but this is really stretching out.

Anyway, a great many IC'ers also have food and substance allergies, and maybe yeast infections to boot, which can also aggravate our problems with allergies and bladder irritation, not to mention our poor little stressed out colons. My colon-bladder-prostate is hurting me right now! If you don't have a prostate, just substitute vulva for the above.

(**Editor note<2014>:** Just a little aside. I wasn't kidding about the sitting problem. About this time I built a special computer desk, which I still have, btw. The table top came up to my belly button. I did this so I could stand and write. Thank goodness the sitting problem got better later on.)

For end-stage IC'ers as I call them...those of us who have about bottomed out, I don't care how well you get using Dr. Fugazotto, or whoever, you best watch what you eat. We know that for most bad-off IC'ers, " coffee, tea, and chocolate are the foundations of pain. It does indeed seem that your no-no list increases as your IC gets worse.

She mentions swollen fingers...Yep....How about a swollen nose, or burning ears, or even bleeding gums....for me, a sure indicator that I've got some serious IC pains on the way.

She says that she gets relief using Elmiron and Elavil, after having tried just about everything. Also mentioned is irritable bowels and the runnies. Is it not reasonable to assume that the self-same bacteria that cause our bladders problems may also inhabit our guts, or at the very least, trigger substances that cause our diarrhea?

She says,"I don't advocate my specific treatment for everyone, but instead, try to let other sufferers know that they must continue to search for their own solution.—No matter how bad their IC may be now, it is possible for it to get better."

Carol also says that, "It was only after I found a way to stop being a victim that I was able to accept my disease." Three cheers for Carol. If you've ever corresponded with Carol, you've pretty well seen the way I think. Super letter, super girl!

*Welcome Debbie M from down Arlington, TX. way!

*Again, I must thank super supporter, Jan K., San Antonio, TX for the material she has sent me as regards her contacts and studies, and also her super work in letting folks out her way know about the ICD. Due to the limited nature of the ICD, I'm getting in so much stuff from time to time that it's impossible for me to do it total justice, however, this little library I'm building should be good for something one of these days. Thanks to all of you, I'm getting smarter and smarter every day about IC, and I'm doing my best to relay the info.

*Julie C Jackson MS. writes to say that she is having success with Dr. F. Her colon is misbehaving though. Tell me about it. She says that when the colon acts up it also causes wee-wee problems. It's all connected, somehow. Off hand, maybe our problems may go back to killing off the friendly bacteria, or encouraging yeast growth in the gut. Maybe an irritated bowel dumps noxious chemicals into the bladder via the bloodstream. One thing is for sure...whenever I have to go tinkle even more often than usual, I can usually trace it back to an acid condition.

Usually, I don't even realize I have acid tummy. A little Mylanta takes care of me, though too much can cause gut problems later. Also, an untreated acid condition today can freak my bladder 3 days later. OK, OK, I love to input stuff....The ICD could just as well have been called CONNECTIONS, because every time I say something or report something someone else says and you identify with it, we just made a connection, and connections count. Good luck to Julie and keep us posted.

* Dr. Fugazotto promises (cross his heart) to publish or otherwise make available his award winning IC recipe for finding those obnoxious little buggers that eat our bladders, very soon. We wait with full bladders.

*Ah ha! So you think ol Norm has kinda slipped a sprocket, do yah, well, take a listen to this from Beverly C. Windham, ME.... "I'm flat on my back because I tried taking beginners ballet class."

This was a ways back, so I reckon the she's back on her toes by now...(Sorry, heh heh.) Alright, at ease, at ease.... So, anyway, Beverly has tried Slippery Elm by now, I reckon. That was my first introduction to the healing arts, as told to me by a gal from Australia. Didn't work long, but it did work, thus showing me that it was possible to improve my condition. She says that she's been eating organic foods too. Let us know how it's coming. Well, I've pecked myself into a corner for sure, so I'll try now to divert your attention to someone else while I try to get back in good graces with Beverly.

*Did I welcome Kaila W from VA onboard last time? Well, welcome aboard anyway.

*The ICD wants to thank Celia L, Phoenix, AZ and the rest of the AZ bunch for some mighty fine work on behalf of all of us. AZ as well as TX are the two newest, and might I say, most enthusiastic supporters of the ICD, and they keep me well informed on what's going on in their neck of the forest. AZ, in particular is doing some great stuff with DR. Fugazotto's work.

Heck, I just hope the VA gang and the AZ gang are pooling their efforts some. The ICD's guess is that from fired up IC'ers like these, great things will come. Remember, you heard it here first. If you want the latest in amateur IC research, you might best get aholt, (As my ol'buddy, Carrie H. from Six Foot would put it) of Celia today.

*Note...... URINARY RESEARCH CENTER, PAUL FUGAZOTTO. Send your wee here after checking with him first. He's good foh what ails you. Oops. I was just congratulating myself on how much text I was squeezing into this issue when I looked up and noticed that I was only on page 7 and a half, and with more mail to go at that. Well, I'll just save that extra page and a half and we'll take up where I left off next time, plus the mail I wasn't able to get to, plus the mail that comes in, in the meantime.

(Editor note<2014>: Yes, I realize that my writing style was terribly corny, but the ladies mostly loved it. I'm guessing now, but it's a safe bet that when my prose became light hearted, it was a sign that my IC wasn't kicking me so badly. Isn't this about the same with you? When your IC is flaring terribly, you're grumpy, and when it lets up a bit, you get a little giddy? The fact is that I was so used to being in dreadful pain that at the rare times I wasn't, I almost missed it. A fact!)

Reckon there's some way that I could have said all that in a shorter manner? The fact is that every once in awhile, I feel kinda cheated. Know what? I look at the pictures of our guys and gals over in Saudi and think to myself, where in the heck is the bathroom. Much is denied us. Every Federal building has a ramp for wheelchairs, but how many have handy bathrooms? In my case, I am fortunate, because my work buddies are ungoshly understanding, much more so than I would be, probably.

I am indeed, legend at the hallowed halls of my company. I tell them that I can take a tinkle faster than they can unzip...and prove it. There's got to be some word for a tinkle artist like myself. I can deplete my bladder in places where it's so crowded you can't even find a seat. Of course, I don't deliberately get myself into these jams. Every single time I see a large crowd, like a rally on TV, I automatically start looking to the sides for the bathrooms.

I can't even remember how it used to be. They say that whenever you lose a body part, your others get stronger. Danged if I've ever found anything that got better about me. But, then again, it could always be worse. You don't ever get used to it, but you have to come to terms with it.

One thing that can help a lot is reducing the pain. Simply put, my advice is to try Dr. Fugazotto, and watch what you eat. Learn your body, and learn to put yourself on a three day study cycle. What you eat today can mess with you now, or at any point in the tubes on its way out. Don't be afraid to try new cures, within reason, and know when to quit. Pain is a good indicator.

What works for one may not work for you, and may even do harm. Getting in tune with your own body will put you way ahead of the game. We've got a long way to go, but we've come a long way, just in the last couple of years. Lean on your support group.

Support the XXX. If you don't like something they are doing, let them know! They are still our best bet; let's just make sure we hedge it a bit. And, for heavens sake, keep the ICD informed on what's happening. God bless till next...NM.

This is an authorized back issue of the ICD reduced to simple ASCII format designed to be read by your word processor. The seemingly errant characters were actually formatting symbols used with the original word processor to enhance the print out. Please try to disregard them as you read this back copy. This is a free service of the ICDisclaimer. All we ask is that if you make use of it, please drop Norman a note that you downloaded it. The original copy, for use with the C-64 and WW5 is available upon request. Norman

The IC Disclaimer Issue 15

(**Editor note<2002>:** This issue ran earlier in the set, but I thought it would be a nice way to end the series here on the net.)

(**Editor note<2014>:** Please recall that in 2002 I edited all of the issues I still had and stashed them for safe keeping on one of my websites. Actually, it was and still is about Brazil travel, a business I used to own. With a little diligent searching it was findable on the search engines of the day. But I chose not to make a mission of it. I had a lot going on at the time and I wasn't prepared to go get back into the IC information business. Already been there and done that. Besides, by this time the Internet had grown up and others had taken up the torch.

Well, times change. In 2014 it was either put the ICD into a book or into the trash can. I chose the former. In 2002 and in 1990 I could not have dreamed of the ease of publishing opportunities to come. A much better solution for the body of the ICD text than a website!)

THE IC DISCLAIMER THE BIMONTHLY NEWSLETTER FOR INTERSTITIAL CYSTITIS YOUR EDITOR: NORMAN MORRISON

THIS MONTH: "BASICS"

This edition of the ICD will be devoted to rooting out the history and nature of Interstitial Cystitis. My information comes primarily from Edward M. Messing writing in the fifth edition of Campbell's Urology, W.B. Saunders and Company, Philadelphia, 1986.

* It appears, from the work of Messing that the notion of IC by one name or another has been around since 1907 when it was recognized by Nitze. Subsequently, several other young gentleman "discovered" the malady, naming it various things. Try, Bladder Fissure,(1939), or cystitis infiltranscircumscripta, (1929), or perhaps good ol' circumscribed panmural ulcerative cystitis, (1920).

It is sometimes described as Hunners Ulcer, a term I'm sure you've heard that goes back to the work of Hunner around 1914.

- Today, Messing describes IC as a syndrome. "This syndrome is defined by the triad of chronic, unexplained irritative voiding symptoms; sterile, cytologically negative urine; and characteristic cystoscopic findings......documentation of all three must be made before a diagnosis of interstitial Cystitis can be established."

So.....from one of the definitive texts of our time you can see that you have a syndrome and that if you fall outside the three criteria even a little bit you have something other than IC, at least that's the way I read it, and I think that's the way your doctor reads it.

Your doctor will more often turn to the work of Messing than Morrison. One thing that clearly puts Messing and Morrison and everybody else with an opinion in the same ball park is that this definitive work is largely. . . .opinion.

(**Editor note<2014>:** And still is. Go look it up on Google. As of this writing all major centers of knowledge can describe it, same as one hundred years ago, but nowhere will you find the cause or cure. Lots of brainy opinions, many of them derived at great cost.)

I certainly hope I did not burst anyone's balloon with this finding. Another observation, is that throughout the years, there have been tight little knots of researchers involved in exploring the IC phenomenon, and that the practical benefits of say, Hunner, has proved about as useful as the work of Messing.

Folks, we have a long way to go, and a short time to get there. In trying to shed a little light on IC, by using Campbell's Urology as source material, I think we'll be a little closer to seeing what your doctor has available.

According to Messing, it is hard to define the incidence of IC, historically, but a late study done in Helsinki in 1975 is deemed most accurate. There, it was found that IC was present in 1.8% of females per 10,000. Other than this, no major studies have been completed which could compare such things as age, race, allergies, etc. to my knowing, except perhaps the poll taken by the XXX a couple of years ago, and I don't have that information.

As Messing says, IC generally takes about 3 to 5 years to progress and stabilize. Even at its worst, it in itself is not life threatening. I might add that there have also been no studies showing what the IC condition might lead to such as cancer, or other problems because of the chronically irritated bladder region, not to mention vulvitis in women and prostatitis in men, with assorted other associated(at least by me) bowel and urinary problems.

Messing notes...."For over 50 years, urologists have been impressed that particular personality traits are common to many patients with (IC)..."

Further,"...we suggest that neurotic traits are more a response to this chronic debilitating condition than its cause."

Messing wisely points to the severe symptoms, long diagnosis times, and reactions of frustrated physicians as perhaps being more the cause for brain problems among the afflicted that we sometimes see, or maybe even exhibit.

My friends, my friends......a person who can not plan more than 15 minutes ahead at a time sometimes has different priorities than regular twice a day people. We're still positive, (I hope), we believe in God, or something, for the most part, and we like children and certain animals. But have you ever wished you could have the power to afflict some pompous TV minister, or maybe some young thing crying because she found a little cellulite on her thighs, just for a couple of hours?

Are you as sympathetic as you used to be? Are you more of a realist now? Are you as patient with what you perceive to be petty aches and pains of others? Are you as patient with doctors as you once were?

You have no doubt read of the GAG layer. You can call it the glycosaminoglycans layer for short. The theory here is that this layer which resides on the luminal surface of the bladder's transitional epithelium (I read this as surface of the bladder lining...correct me if I'm wrong) acts as a protective agent. Liken it to a downhill racer wearing a diving wetsuit. If he falls, he'll just slide on down the hill, whereas without it he'd just by and by turn into one big rash by the time he hits bottom.

Likewise, this layer may serve to keep bacteria, or perhaps even pesky little urea crystals (you can see them under a microscope) away from the meaty portion of the bladder. Messing was not sold on this theory, therefore neither would the physician who uses his text as a guide...see, we can find some "roots" if we look hard enough.

Messing touches on one of my favorite areas, and says, "To our knowledge, investigations in these directions have not been pursued."

We concern ourselves now with urine, and toxic substances which may abound there. Obviously, folks, our urine is contacting the deeper layers of the bladder and just shriveling it on down. We experience referred pain at the head of the penis if we happen to have one, or in the vulvular region if we drew one of those. The bottom of our feet hurt and we have gastrointestinal problems, all stemming, or working in conjunction with the bladder.

We all have the funky, mostly useless shriveled bladder in common. Do we have weak bladder or perhaps regular bladder and potent pee pee?

The area of urine-analysis research is virgin territory. Notice, I did not say urinalysis, which is what you get when you go to the doc. He looks for bacteria, blood, and white blood cells. If he's uptown, he may check for sugar and albumen, and a couple of other things. No, I'm talking about a sure-enough-bonafide study of the normal person's urine as versus the urine produced by the IC sufferer.

IF we could find some differences, we'd be a lot closer to finding the proper avenue to base all of our research. In other words, are we producing toxic substances that help us to eat ourselves up?

One of our main problems in IC research is pulling the various scientific disciplines together. I'm sure that there is already a great body of research out there on the components of urine. No doubt, studying stomach ulcers could shed light on the factors that enable IC.

We know, you and I, that studying unrelated research on allergies have helped us to eat smarter and avoid IC causing foods like chocolate, coffee, and tea. Are there acids or proteins in the foods that we know universally affect

IC folks? If so, what are they? I only know of one thing that comes into contact with the bladder wall with regularity, and that is urine. This of course brings us back to the chicken/egg argument. Did our bladder shrink up first, or did the urine shrink the bladder up.

At the least, I think that our urine may hold one heck of a lot of answers, and that studying related areas of research such as ulcers could be helpful. We may already have a lot of answers right there on the shelf if we can find the right person to just stretch right up and pluck it down.)

Messing states, "Patients will often be told that they have other urologic diseases." (There are good plumbers as well as bad ones.)

He also states once again, "Cultures are invariably sterile, since the diagnosis of [IC] cannot be made in the face of bacterial, fungal, mycobacterial, chlamydial, parasitic, gonococcal, or other infections."

Is the good doctor saying that folks with IC cannot suffer from the above afflictions? It looks like it to me. As you know, our weakened constitutions lend us to all sorts of urologic problems, and when we get one, it's the devil getting rid of it. How many people have been called IC free just because they had the misfortune to also have a persistent bacterial infection at diagnosis time?

How many IC victims have been treated for a "real bad" yeast infection? And so it goes.

Diagnosing IC is an easy and rewarding pastime. If you are as healthy as an astronaut, except for the otherwise tedious gnawing in your groin, the procedure called Hydrodistension is indicated.

Messing suggests that the bladder be pumped up to a working pressure of 70cm of water. Cystoscopic examination reveals a normal or nearly normal bladder in folks whose bladder can hold 450cc or more of fluid. End stage IC'ers who have teeny bladders, (under 400cc capacity) show scarring immediately.

Otherwise, the fluid is drained, showing a little blood in the last little bit, and pumped up again. This time, glomerulations appear and IC can be readily diagnosed. Clearly, here, you see that there is a marked difference between those of us who are just coming down with IC and those of us who have had it awhile, with the severely reduced bladder capacity to show for it.

For long time IC folks, the doctor can expect to see copious amounts of blood the first time around. Thankfully, the patient must be under an anesthetic, so that the bladder muscles will relax to allow for maximum distention, otherwise, the doctor himself might be severely bloodied by the patient.

There are many, many treatments available for the typical IC sufferer, unfortunately, most are weird and don't work. Presently, we battle, virtually alone, except for one another of us, as has the problem, trying various approaches, ranging from watching our diet to crying a lot. Some of us have our bladder taken out; some have a little intestine added.

Sometimes we try a little shot of horse liniment, or a steroid or two. Invariably, we just survive.

I personally feel that the answer is in front of our face....we just haven't yet seen it. Too many of us have too much in common (like allergies) that you wouldn't normally associate with IC. One of these days a budding Pasteur out there is going to find that magic bullet. We have to do it!

The thing that makes the ICD tick is the mail, of course! You keep me smiling. One thing I didn't count on was getting more money than I asked for. Two of my great IC buddies, Pat S in Georgia and AJ over in Wisconsin sent in more than the required amount. By the time I heard from Pat, Alice had already sent in a couple of checks. She really had me scratching my head, so I was prepared, if not quite humbled.

These extra gifts will allow me to get some professional looking envelopes,(as quickly as managing editor, my wife, Vicky) gets around to it. Also, it will help me break even, which is all I want to do, since I'm just po' folks.

****(Please note, this little aside is in praise of my friends. Your six bucks was all I asked for and MUCH appreciated too!) Happily, I checked with the federal government, (THEY know what's best for us.) and it will be some time before I should have to worry about the tax situation. You must make over $400.00 in a little enterprise like this before having to even report your income. Since the ICD is not for profit but taxable just the same it will be awhile yet before our budget gets that high.

You might be interested to know that we have about 20 subscribers so far, many of them in some of the most influential XXX positions, just outside the inner circle. I'm more than tickled for you to reprint as much of the ICD as you'd like, just as long as you include the disclaimer at the top, or something indicating that we too say, "See your doctor."

The low but growing number of subscribers belies the fact that a lot of folks are seeing copies and snips of the ICD. Thanks to you. I hope you will continue to see something here and there in the ICD that you think will do your friends good! Talk about a shot in the arm. AJ , with the Wisconsin gang is hereby promoted to GUARDIAN ANGEL. I get around two letters a month, and a whole lot of support from this nice person.

AJ met with Dr. Crook (the allergist) at the end of April and had a battery of tests. She is allergic to most everything, about like you would expect. I'll let you know how she progresses under Dr. Crook's care. You might want to see him yourself someday.

*****Last issue, I premiered the SLP Database. Well, exit the SLP Database until we get a few more subscribers. One of the foremost reasons for having the thing was to help and identify allergens common to most of us. Why re-invent the wheel? It just so happens that there is already such a list of foods available, and I got no less than three copies of it in the mail.

The ICD believes in the importance of staying away from certain foods. Most happily, I already knew about a good many of the foods on this list....the hard way. This leads me to believe that I'm on the right track after all. I appreciate your prompt response in this area. One of the respondees was Pat S. In addition to the list she writes that she is using Elavil and following Larrian <Gillespie's> advice in the book, "You Don't Have To Live With Cystitis."

Also, Pat recommends 1 teaspoon of baking soda in a glass of water followed later on in the day by some other antacid such as Tums for tummy acid which gives your bladder jumping fits. Pat says that tea made using the SUN TEA method is OK. Now, Pat, I'm dubious, but by golly I'm going to risk my poor old bladder and give it a try. I used to live on the boiled stuff, and as a southerner, I'm mostly lost without it. Here's looking at you, kid. Let me just quickly list those foods that you should avoid like the plague. Of course, there are exceptions to every rule.....

All alcoholic beverages(some late harvest wines excepted), apples, apple juice, cantaloupe, carbonated beverages, cherries, chili spices, cumin, ginger, Hungarian paprika, chutney, curry, citrus fruits, coffee, cranberries, grapes, guava, lemon juice, papaya, peaches, pickles, watermelon rind, persimmons, pineapple, rhubarb, pomegranate, strawberries, tea, tomatoes, vinegar, avocados, bananas, beer, brewers yeast, canned figs, champagne, cheese, (ceptin processed cheeses such as Velveeta, ricotta, mozzerella, cream cheese, string cheese, and cottage cheese.), chicken livers, chocolate, (ceptin carob or white....((maybe)), corned beef, eggplant, fava beans, lima beans, mayonaise, Nutrasweet, nuts, onions, pickled herring, prunes, raisins, rye bread, Sacchrine, sour cream, soy sauce, Worstershire sauce, yougart, and some vitamins..............

Larrian developed the original list, and I'm sure that you will have your own additions and deletions to add to the list.

IF I had this list two or three years ago I could have saved myself much pain! Again, thanks for sending it in.

The IC DISCLAIMER is non-profit, but not tax deductible. One year costs $6.00. It is published 6 times a year. Please make your check payable to: Norman Morrison, the editor of this magazette. .... Back issues are available at regular prices. Write. THANKS!

All correspondence is considered public unless you specify otherwise. Your address may be made available to others with similar interests unless you say otherwise. KEEP WRITING!

How do you tell if you are allergic to something? That's the question a young lady posed to me a while back. Here's how I do it. Suppose, for example that I suspect that cheese on the 99 cent Booger Doodle Cheesyburger I like so well is doing a number on my bladder. I simply go out and get, (if my wife will spring for it and go get....) a big hunk of that delicious hoop cheese, (or whatever serves for a lot of cheese in your locale) and make sure that I dine on it like a pig on cake.

Shake, and wait 2 to 4 days. If I get worse, I'll lay off for a few days, then pig out again. After 3 or 4 delicious interludes I'll know whether or not I'll ever have another one.

I find that you can have a little of some foods, by and by and mostly get away with it. Others will convulse your tinkle center after just a whiff. Try it, you may like it!

I have been blessed with some SUPER newsletters. Let me extend my thanks to each and every person who was so thoughtful. Actually, some of them kinda put the ICD format in the shade. Pro jobs all! First in the out batch comes one from Ruth K in Fairfax, Va. They are doing some GREAT things up there. They just had a guest who is a local Elmiron researcher and were looking forward to a meeting with another gentleman who reportedly has developed a souped up test for allergies. Perhaps Ruth will share any results that she feels may be of use to her ICD friends out of state. Ruth also sends an address for the NATIONAL CHRONIC PAIN OUTREACH ASSOCIATION, INC., <Address>. Should you contact these folks, let the ICD know how it went.

Also, (Jan J.) and others, Ruth sends this address—Food and Nutrition Information Center, National Agricultural Library, <Address>. This is a good address to tuck away for those of you who are interested in food/substances connections, like how much tannic acid you'll get in a glass of tea.

Finally, one last eye opener...Ruth lets it be known that low acid tomatoes may not be so low in acid after all. Ruth says that varieties that are 4.5ph or higher are safe to munch. Among them, Beefmaster Hybrid, Ace55VF, Big Early Hybrid, Big Girl, Burpee VF Hybrid, Delicious, but NOT Better Boy.....shucks! Thanks for this chunk of info Ruth!!!

I work on the weekends, so most XXX type stuff is strictly off limits. I especially hate that when I get newsletters like the one from The GEORGIA "GOTTA GO" GROUP. Their newsletter is a truly professional job. Nita H, Lori M, and good ol' Bill O, head the team for the Georgia effort.

There wasn't a lot of hard info in this issue because they are just getting started. I especially wanted you to know what a great job this dedicated young team is doing. Please to keep the ICD on your mailing list. Pray for their success.

Holly L, the Wisconsin Coordinator sends her regards and some much needed information to the ICD. The editor thanks her to the fullest, as he has not been able to come up with said info elsewhere. Among some of the printables, Holly notes that she is a multi-sufferer. OH? I thought that IC folks just had sterile urine and hurt down there some?

I shall steal the term multi-sufferer for future use. Holly says that she suffered FOCAL VULVITIS, also known as VULVODYNIA. (Sounds sort of like what Russians drink to my untrained ear.) I have had several folks comment on this. In your letters in the future, you might wish to comment on this condition as it relates to IC and we'll focus on it in a future issue.

In the meantime, Holly characterizes it thusly, "Vulvodynia involves chronic vulvar pain and burning to various degrees, and/or vulvar itching, tenderness at entrance of vagina, and usually involves lesions in the vestibule that are extra sensitive and painful to the touch, and most often severe enough to make intercourse impossible. A number of studies and articles are available."

This, of course, is not to be confused with vaginitis. Holly's newsletter is excellent, and the Wisconsin folks are indeed lucky to have her. By now, she should be at the Kenneth Norris Jr. Cancer Hospital at USC in Los Angeles having a Koch pouch procedure. I'm sure she could use your encouragement. I'm not sure of the address there, but I'm sure that she would still get your mail if you want to send her a card or what. Her address is: Holly L, Menomonie, WI .

She sent me a clipping from her local paper, and it looks like the whole town is pulling for her! We are too.

(Editor note<2014>: Remember, this was an earlier edition that I moved to the end of the stack because as I noted in 2002, it just seemed to fit. Below, the introduction to Dr. Fugazotto, who will become very important in the life of the ICD.)

A note of interest. In the mail, we learn of a new avenue of attack on IC. First, from Melanie B, and then from Ruth K, news came in about a gentleman called, Paul Fugazzotto, MSPH,PhD. After a talk with the good <fellow?> I can report that I believe that he believes in his program, although it goes somewhat contrary to current wisdom. (Our kind of guy.)

To explain, as briefly as possible, Dr. F. has come up with a better way of identifying micro-organisms. He presented his findings to the XXX and recently before the NIH. He maintains that the standard urinalysis just doesn't work for IC folks. He has found a certain kind of infection that is common to most IC'ers, and certain patterns.

One of our number has reported possible success with his program, and at least two more semi-reputable folks are guinea pigging and trying the cure, (myself included.)

In my case, I'm simply taking Nystatin,(The standby yeast medicine) and an antibiotic that isn't normally on the IC list. Simply put, Dr. F. believes that IC is caused by the bacteria you haven't found. Get it? IC caused from bacterial infection.

The consensus is, I think, "It sounds too good to be true." Well, we'll see. If you are on the program, for heavens sake, let me know your progress. If you want more information, you can reach the doc thusly: Paul Fugazzotto, <address> . He's a real nice guy, and will I'm sure he will answer your questions. I hope against hope that this proves to be a viable approach, since it's minimal in risk, but like I told the doctor, the ICD for sure needs to see results before reaching anything approaching a conclusion. There are many more items that we could touch on, but there comes a time to end. My phone number, by the way, is (X). Its best to catch me on Thursday thru Sunday evenings.

Until we meet again, just remember...things could always be worse. Be thankful for what you have. The next issue will wind up the first year of the ICD, thanks to you. I think it's been a pretty good year. God bless, all. Norman

This ends the ICD portion of this book.

Regarding Dr. Paul Fugazzotto, Ph.D.

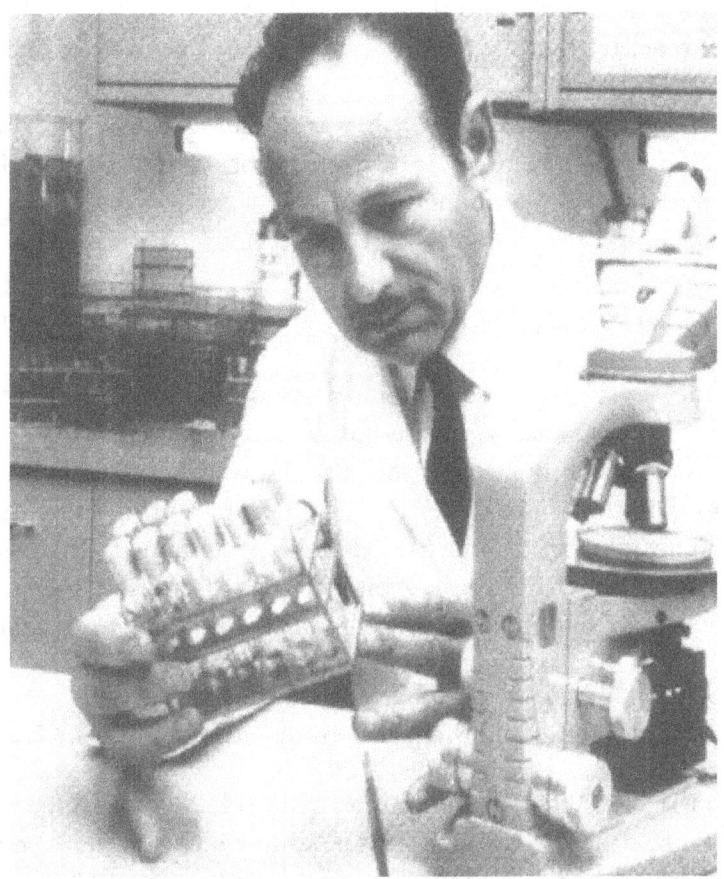

Photo reproduced by permission of owner. Dr. Paul Fugazzotto at work.

The photo above is of Dr. Paul Fugazzotto, Ph.D in his younger years. Dr. F. for short. This chapter of the Pioneers of IC is dedicated to him.

According to a web page provided by a funeral home, "Dr. Paul Fugazzotto, 95, died at the Rapid City Regional Auxiliary Hospice House on Wednesday, Aug. 6, 2008. He was born on March 20, 1913, in Newburgh, N.Y., the son of Sicilian immigrants."

As you have seen in the ICD, Dr. F. took up quite a bit of space. He was one of the leading characters in the evolution of my thinking on the matter. He made his first appearance in the ICD in issue 6.

Fundamental is that you must understand that I and my readers knew that Interstitial Cystitis stems from a bacterial infection after Dr. F. explained it to us. Further proof came from Dr. Rosalind Maskell over in England. You can find a ton of references to her on Google.

I was quite excited when I was made aware of Maskell, after studying the work of Fugazzotto. At the time it seemed that a slam dunk was in progress in that we had two independent and different proofs of the bacterial cause of IC.

I was in for a rude lesson. The other, better known and more famous researchers of the day, busy with their interesting but dead end experiments refused to take notice of the cause of IC right in front of their noses. I likened the work of Dr. F. to a Paul Muni movie, wherein he was Pasteur and the other guys were the ones at the science institute ridiculing those mythical microbe things. How could something you couldn't see make you sick? Ridiculous!

I'm not joking. That's how I came to view it and that is how it was.

Worst of all Dr. F. didn't act like he cared. He steadfastly refused to publish his work in the fancy medical magazines. That eventually burned me. I could not understand.

Well, time, age, and wisdom come along and I was finally able to reconcile the odd things going on about me. Two things: First, Dr. F. refused to jump into the publishing rat race. But secondly, I had lost most respect for the research system as I came to believe that the IC research of the day wasn't so much about IC as just...research into interesting things.

Put more simply, it appeared that while Dr. F. was searching for the cure, his counterparts were busy trying to understand the effects. This is two completely different things. One leads to relief and the other leads to semi-interesting scientific papers and more grant money.

As it turned out Dr. F. and I were in total agreement about the whole publish and get a grant dog and pony show... I just didn't realize it at the time.

Time passes. More than twenty years. I decide to publish a book about the Pioneers of IC and one of the first things I look for in preparation is an update on Dr. F.

Luckily for me I knew what city his son lived in and his approximate profession. Google supplied the rest of the information necessary for me to be able to locate and contact him.

With no expectation of a reply one way or the other I was surprised and pleased when he called me.

As it turns out, son David was just a week or so away from retiring from his physician job at a busy medical center. Without a doubt in my mind the timing MUST mean something. If I had waited a week, the opportunity of reaching him would have been much harder, as he is on an extended vacation, even as I write this.

As it turned out he published not one, but two books by his father, posthumously, in 2008...

1. Pelvic Disorder: Stirring Adventures of the Medical Detective
2. Laboratory Manual In Diagnosis and Management of Pelvic Disorders: Cystitis

Both books are copyright 2008 by Paul Fugazzotto MSPH, Ph.D

David published both, either by a vanity press or simply ordering more copies as he needs them somehow. They are not public domain. I advised him of the self publishing system, of which you are using now and I hope he makes use of it in the future.

The books were news to me. Very very welcome news. In *Pelvic Disorder: Stirring Adventures of the Medical Detective* Dr. F. has all the fun with his remarkable biography and gives 62 case studies where his microbial detective work solved everything from crimes to laboratory mysteries.

The books by Dr. F. elaborate on what is written in The IC Disclaimer Issue 7. In *Pelvic Disorder: Stirring Adventures of the Medical Detective* Dr. F. states unequivocally, "The CC is an absolute fraud." Then he systematically goes about showing why this is so.

"CC" refers to what he calls the "classic culture" technique of urine that has been in place for the last half century. It's what I describe in detail in the ICD.

Shortly, when your urine goes to the lab using the classic culture technique, the clinicians are looking for a grow out of pathogenic harmful bacteria in a pre-ordained quantity. This rarely if ever happens with the classic methods employed, thus your physician gets a report of negative growth. In the ICD days that most often meant a shrug of the shoulders or possibly a round of antibiotics on a guess. You can't treat what's not there. Women were often accused of simply being nuts.

Dr. F., on the other hand did not look for a colony count of bacteria, per se. He searched for whatever he found, and when he scored, no matter the colony count, he knew he had the perpetrator.

Finding IC causing pathogens is not possible with the factory CC method. As Dr. F. demonstrated you first need to find a way to grow out bacteria that don't normally multiply using established methods, and then you need to get out the microscope and actually look at them.

You know when you think about IC for about five minutes you can see the cleverness of Dr. F.s thinking. IC isn't something with no known cause or cure. Something is definitely causing it and when you find out what it is, then there may well be a cure. It's just common every day good walking around sense that has managed to elude the egg headed so called IC researchers for decades.

In the summary of the introduction of *Pelvic Disorder: Stirring Adventures of the Medical Detective* Dr. F. states, "The approach of the medical detective is directed by the age old universal rule of Cause & Effect: where there is a <u>disorder</u> there is also an effective <u>cause</u>, and the detective must have the integrity and obligation to resolve the matter to a decisive conclusion."

As a practical example, think back to your visit to the doctor. If a sample of urine was given, how long did it take the doctor to report a clear culture? By comparison Dr. F.'s methods takes days, and sometimes repeat samples. He was not looking for a certain count of proscribed bacteria. He looked for whatever he could find. Sometimes even he was surprised at what turned up in the "clear" sample. More on this shortly.

Dr. F. fondly referred to himself as a "microbe hunter." He was never more happy than when, with microscope in hand, on the stalk for wily, lurking bacteria. He had little patience with clinicians who go about their jobs by rote. He advocated always that the laboratory technician must proceed with imagination and integrity. He reckoned it was his job to give the doctor the correct findings, even if it wasn't what the doctor expected.

In his book, *Laboratory Manual In Diagnosis and Management of Pelvic Disorders: Cystitis* Dr. F. gives his complete recipe for the culture of IC causing microorganisms that traditional techniques cannot find. He also discusses the antibiotics that are useful in the treatment.

You know, if the world gets nothing else from his books, which would be a shame, the formula for culturing the pathogenic bugs that cause our IC is priceless.

Back in the ICD days I knew generally how he went about his work. He wasn't one to keep secrets. However, the exact recipe, if you will, was not published in a way that only a trained microbiologist could use to decipher his technique.

Since, I have seen a version of it on the Internet on an old website, which is suspect. His book, however spells it out.

I would like to quote from the book a passage that you will find interesting as an armchair urologist. Keep in mind that while Dr. F. was a superior microbiologist, he spoke and wrote in language that the laymen, such as you and I would understand...

The Principles of Cardinal Diagnostic Rules

1. All infections are SYMPTOMATIC, and due to their specific pathogen.

2. Normal human strains of *Escherichia coli,* are not pathogens. They are strict saprophytes with no pathogenic quality.

3. There is <u>no disease entity diagnosed on the basis of bacterial numbers.</u> The etiologic agents must be recognized by the trained laboratorian for their <u>pathogenic cultural characteristics as infectious agents.</u>

4. In all case the RULE OF CAUSE & EFFECT assures that where there is a disorder there is a related CAUSE, the identity of which is essential to the clinician's appraisal of the patient's condition; and must be reported to the clinician for the patient's treatment.

5. Medical schools recognize raw urines as agglomerations of body wastes, which may antagonize the emergence of pathogens. Use of scavenger saprophytes is an erroneous layman concept, and a violation of the pioneers established Cardinal Diagnostic Rules.

6. In tests of urine, to assure that all strains present do emerge for evaluation, primary culture must be made in general purpose broth, followed by transfer to differential media for isolation and identification of the causative pathogen.

7. The identity of a disease is determined by use of differential media for isolating and identifying its etiologic agent.

8. In keeping with the principles of Hippocrates, organisms infecting tissues of the upper body may be expected to transmigrate by way of the bloodstream to the kidneys and urine, as well as those ascending from fecal contamination of the perineum.

Once you digest the bulk of Dr. F.'s diagnostic rules, of particular interest is the last entry here. *Urine is never sterile.* It's pretty darned interesting, to me, at least, that bacterial organisms from elsewhere in the body can invade and live in the bladder environment. When you give this a bit of thought, it is not outlandish at all. The human body plays host to all sorts of weird flora. Why should the bladder be a critter free zone?

Keep in mind that when someone visits the doctor's office with a simple case of cystitis, the problem is quickly identified and dealt with. When you, on the other hand, stop by with your case, the doctor finds no evidence of infection, unless you also happen to have a bout of the regular garden variety cystitis as well.

Dr. F.'s rule, is that when someone came to him in pain, there is cause and effect, and a reason for it. Saying that a patient must be ok because they beat all the regular tests was never an option for him. He kept dogging it until he came up with an answer. This is what he demands of modern clinicians. If the patient dodges all the handy tests, then come up with a new one.

This is good advice, in general, for all us IC'ers. Just because we fail at regulating our pain using the tried and true methods, we must never stop searching. We are sick. There is a cause. Find the cause and treat the condition.

Trigger Mechanism

At this point I need to make something clear. For Interstitial Cystitis to occur there must be three things present:

1. A host.

2. A pathogenic organism.

3. A trigger.

Dr. F. called point three a *trigger mechanism*. The trigger mechanism is what makes IC so damnably hard to get our heads around. Since the ICD days I have explained that there is no doubt in my mind that most people play host to the same kind of misery causing germs as we do, but they never get IC. Why?

Dr. F. seems to agree with me straight from the grave. He noted, for instance, that childbirth is a fantastic time for a woman to acquire IC. First time sex in the female is another.

But beyond that, in your own case, can you recall something out of the ordinary around the time of onset? A trauma? Stress? Injury? A sickness of some kind?

In my case, my main suspect is that I was on a no carbohydrate diet when I first noticed a burning bladder. Perhaps the change in my metabolism allowed a confluence of bad luck to open the door to unwanted bladder visitors who took up residence. That's my theory. What's yours?

In conclusion, it is my fond hope that the books of Dr. Paul Fugazzotto will one day be available to the community so you can read for yourself what I have attempted to condense. The books are written in such a way that both the armchair urologist and the hard working microbiologist both will benefit from the pioneering work of this wonderful, kind man who toward the end of his lengthy and illustrious career made it his mission to help those of us afflicted with Interstitial Cystitis.

So what of the future, or perhaps the past, as you read this, of research into the bacterial nature of IC?

In a hand written note from David Fugazzotto that came with my books he happened to mention that PCR techniques were making some inroads to the bacterial infections of the bladder. I had no idea what he was talking about so I went to Google for a look.

According to Wikipedia, PCR is short for *polymerase chain reaction* which has to do with the study of DNA. I do not profess to know any more than this. In our case, the applicable use is, as Wiki says, "...identification of non-cultivatable or *slow-growing microorganisms* such as mycobacteria, anaerobic bacteria, or viruses from tissue culture assays and animal models. The basis for PCR diagnostic applications in microbiology is the detection of infectious agents and the discrimination of non-pathogenic from pathogenic strains by virtue of specific genes."

Recall that Dr. F.'s procedure was all about slow growing, difficult to culture bacteria.

Further investigation led to an article on Medscape entitled *Urine is Not Sterile, PCR Analysis Shows* by Jenni Laidman April 13, 2012.

(http://hsd.luc.edu/newswire/news/loyola-study-debunks-common-myth-urine-sterile)

That's nice. ICD'ers knew that twenty five years ago. (From my perch in good old 2014.)

In my experience this was the third confirmation of the fact. Recall that Fugazzotto and Maskell proved that but were soundly ignored.

This led me to contact the author of the research, an extremely nice fellow, Alan J. Wolfe, PhD, professor of microbiology and immunology, Stritch School of Medicine, Loyola University in Chicago.

From previous experience I really didn't expect a reply, but reply he did the same day!

Wolfe doesn't claim to have found the Holy Grail of IC or anything like that, but I can't help but think that Dr. Fugazzotto would have been extremely interested in this new line of research.

From his lofty position at Loyola University, he's sure to have the credentials to make his colleagues sit up and take notice as his work progresses. Thus, once again, I am hopeful that the research community will finally one day realize that the treatment is far more simple than previously thought.

In the meantime, while I had not set out to make connections, I did. Wolfe was aware of Maskell's work, but Dr. F. was new to him. I managed to hook him up with Dr. F.'s son David. He may learn that history is the future!

The valuable lesson here is to establish leads through diligent research and follow up on them. Make connections. Generate new knowledge. Get proactive in your own personal understanding of Interstitial Cystitis. Nobody, including your doctor and all the research folks have more at stake than you do.

The IC Disclaimer Epilog

I have not visited my copies of the ICD since 2000 or so when I ran it over from whatever format I had it saved to, to something that would look passable on a modern computer. Much of what I read in preparing, I had forgotten. It was like a visit with old friends.

I am the sort of person who tends to remember pleasing things. Therefore, I only generally recall what became of the magazette.

It ran a few more issues than I have here, because they are lost. Generally speaking, by the time I wound it down, I was hurting pretty good (You know the drill) and I had become disillusioned that we'd ever get the problem solved. For my life I don't recall if it was a sudden decision to end the ICD or if it came on gradually. Either way, I closed shop and moved on. By this time I was also co-herd master of a couple of pre-teen children. Also, my father, who I worked with in the family business died. Life definitely got in the way of my magazine editor duties.

If you're curious, I never did find my personal cure for IC. Currently, I'm doing a good bit better than I was in my ICD days. My greatest gains came at the end of my last day job.

I attribute going from what I called "end stage" IC in the ICD to moderate IC to the fact that I have diligently worked to identify and eliminate every substance that I could find that made me hurt. Also, it is possible that as has been reported, occasionally getting older helps. The body, sometimes, is not as keen to destroy itself. Sort of like someone who "grows out" of allergies. It happens.

Stress relief has also played a major part. I can't stress strongly enough that stress will absolutely aggravate IC. It's stressful enough just having to deal with it.

While, on the one hand, I am not in constant pain and going every five minutes like I did for nearly 30 years previously, I have still not experienced anything approaching a full night of sleep since I got the awful stuff. Also, while I may get a bit cocky during the winter, the summer time allergens really wilt my spirit. It's still a struggle to do the things I have to do outside. IC is tiring!

Lastly, there is time itself. While I am doing better than I was, I am getting older. I simply don't have the stamina to fight through flare-ups like I used to. In a different way, my bad days, while not as bad are as draining as they used to be.

So, I have my good days and my bad days. My good days are dedicated to doing whatever I can to have less bad days! Is this about the same with you?

As I mentioned earlier, I brought certain good and important memories from my time with the ICD. Chief among them is that, "What you eat *can* hurt you." The same goes for what you breathe and touch as well.

I also came to understand that in our struggle with IC, less is better than more. Always go for the least invasive treatment you can. There is always time to step it up. If herbs help you, then why risk powerful drugs? If natural remedies fail, you can always get the good stuff from the doctor.

I came to the conclusion that, "If it hurts, don't do it."

This goes for herbs, drugs, pizza, or whatever makes your bladder go ouch. You MUST use YOUR common sense. Never be a doctor worshiper. In the final analysis, nobody knows better how you feel than you. But, on the other hand, don't try to play doctor when it comes to prescription medication like antibiotics. Follow the label instructions. Use it, or don't use it, but don't try to reinvent the wheel. Incorrect antibiotic usage can be worse than none at all.

I know I don't have to remind you that personal research is your main tool to helping yourself with your problem.

You know, if I had not stopped the ICD snail mail magazette, the Internet would have stopped it for me. There are whole libraries more information available to you now than just ten or fifteen short years ago. Frankly, if you don't have the gumption to use what's out there, I really don't have much going for you. Be the armchair urologist. Do your research....and...when you make a discovery, share it with others. Don't be an info hog. Please.

Looking back, I'd say one half of the reason that I discontinued my ground breaking newsletter was that I finally threw in the towel of ever expecting a cure from the big time researchers out there. I'd say, in hindsight that I pretty well nailed that one! I still see no cure.

On the other hand, nearly every method that you use or will use to help alleviate the mind killing pain of your IC was developed by regular, ordinary, unfunded IC sufferers just like you. Baskets and boxcar loads of IC tips and tricks from folks just like you are out there and freely available for you to investigate.

When you get IC, it really comes down to two things. (1), you will lapse into despair and denial and live the life of a victim, easy prey for charlatans and know nothing doctors or (2) you will get fired up, educated, and motivated to do whatever it takes to lick, or at least live with the beast. I have seen it go both ways. I can't help but wonder if the despairing types are even still alive today.

I also learned one truly awful thing that I wish I hadn't. "You can't help the helpless."

Here's the deal. The keys to a better life are out there for IC folks. That being the case, feel sorry for those who CHOOSE NOT to use them, but do not let them drag you down into their pit born of stubbornness leading to unending sorrow. They'll do it, if you let them. Don't. That's just good advice for life in general.

And truly, my friend, never get stigmatized about your urine obsession. Everybody that lives has to go tinkle. It's just that we do it more frequently. If your friends be true, they'll put up with it. Even joke with you about it. A very nice girl who departed a job at which I worked gave presents around before she left. She gave me a t-shirt with a dog, leg hiked, peeing with a splash. In big letters at the top of the drawing it said, "Potty Animal."

You know, it isn't fair that we have to make water all the time and our friends don't. But, it's what we drew when we decided to live on earth. It's just the breaks. We can't live our painful lives with IC *and* urine envy too. Way too much to worry with!

Be of good cheer, even when it hurts. The sorry fact is that what we have could always be worse. Wait. You don't believe me? Ok, I'll prove it. What's worse than your IC right now? How about your IC and a painful paper cut? See? It can always be worse. So rejoice that you're not any worse off than you are. Right? Let me see that smile now. Aha, you're smiling and you don't even want to. Ha! See how easy it is?

We have one thing in common, you and I. We're elite members of a pretty exclusive club. The trick to surviving is to make it a purpose in your life to never stop researching and applying yourself to hurt less. Also, giving back to the IC community which has given to you will ultimately pay off big dividends. Current dividends are running to ten times ten of what you originally put into the system.

Surviving with IC is challenging, but it can be fun and productive as well. It's all in how you approach and deal with the problem.

I'm thinking you're up to the task. So, get off your bladder and get busy making a plan for the rest of your life.

One final piece of ICD business...

As always, your reviews of this book here where you purchased it are always welcome. Reviews make a difference, thumbs up or thumbs down.

But beyond that, especially if you happen to be a dear former reader of the ICD, it would be great if you would take time to pen a note in the *comments* here (if provided), identify yourself, and tell everyone how you have progressed since the pioneering ICD days. (Yes, I know this isn't an IC forum, but you'll have to admit it will get seen a lot by IC'ers.)

And, naturally, if you have wonderful new armchair research to impart, PLEASE do! That, my friend, would be VERY nice indeed! (New ICD readers also invited to participate.) Carry on, fellow IC'ers!

Take care and thanks for spending time with me and the ICD!
Norman Morrison
IC'er since 1982 (Resigned but never defeated!)